YOUR QUESTIONS,
YOUR CONCERNS,
YOUR RIGHT
TO GOOD HEALTH ...

We have written this book to help our readers identify previously unrecognized thyroid problems in themselves or among their relatives and friends. For some, it may serve as a guide to proper medical attention and treatment. We hope other readers will simply enjoy it as an introduction to a fascinating part of the remarkable body in which we live.

We have also written this book in the hope that it will reflect a new and refreshing attitude toward medical care in general. You as a patient have the *right* as well as the responsibility to know what is going on when you get sick—to know the cause of your illness, what tests or treatments you should have, why they are necessary, and what the course of your illness is likely to be. Health education of this type is important because it enables you to play a more helpful part in the care of your own body, and that in itself should help you to be a healthier person.

YOUR THYROID
A HOME
REFERENCE

3rd Edition

Lawrence C. Wood, M.D., F.A.C.P.
David S. Cooper, M.D., F.A.C.P.
E. Chester Ridgway, M.D., F.A.C.P.

BALLANTINE BOOKS • NEW YORK

We dedicate this Third Edition to our children

    LCW: Peter, Ty, Marianna
    ECR: Emily, Eli, Abby
    DSC: Jonathan, Ethan, Susanna

Copyright © 1982, 1995 by Lawrence C. Wood, M.D.

All rights reserved under International and Pan-American Copyright Conventions. Published in the United States by Ballantine Books, a division of Random House, Inc., New York, and simultaneously in Canada by Random House of Canada Limited, Toronto. Originally published in a different form by Ballantine Books in 1982.

Library of Congress Catalog Card Number: 82-6494

ISBN 0-345-39170-5

Printed in Canada

First Mass Market Edition: December 1986
Third Edition: July 1995

10 9 8 7 6

Contents

PREFACE

We wrote this book for you

- *If you are struggling with an overactive or underactive thyroid—and don't know it.* There are nearly eight million such people in the United States alone, and there are good treatments for both conditions when they are recognized.

- *If any of your close relatives has a goiter or has been treated for a thyroid disorder.* Many thyroid problems run in families, and maybe you should be checked too.

- *If you have an overactive thyroid, you may have older relatives who have a failing thyroid.* They, along with younger members of your family, should have their thyroids tested.

- *If you are pregnant.* Thyroid problems are extremely common during the year following delivery. A simple blood TSH test can help you and your doctor tell if your thyroid malfunctions.

- *If you had neck irradiation in childhood during X-ray treatment for a condition such as acne, tonsillitis, or an enlarged thymus gland.* Your risk for benign and cancerous thyroid tumors is increased (most thyroid cancers can be cured).

- *If you are concerned about the potential health risks of a nuclear-reactor accident.* Radioactive iodine released by such an event could lead to thyroid problems.

- *If you were treated for a thyroid problem in the past.* We now know that many thyroid problems need lifelong attention.

- *If you are taking thyroid pills for overweight, infertility, sluggishness, or depression.* Your treatment probably needs to be reviewed and updated.

- *If you are facing a test, medical treatment, or operation for your thyroid.* This book will tell you what it means and what it will be like.

- *If you are taking or thinking of taking kelp.* The iodine in kelp could make a lumpy thyroid dangerously overactive. If you are pregnant, it could make your unborn baby's thyroid enlarge or fail.

- *If you are concerned about the possibility of a nuclear accident occurring near your home.* There is radioactive iodine in fallout that could have harmful effects on your thyroid unless you take a small amount of nonradioactive iodine to protect your thyroid.

- *If you take insulin for diabetes, need vitamin B12 for anemia, have prematurely gray hair, or have white skin patches known as vitiligo.* Your risk for an overactive or underactive thyroid may be increased, and perhaps your thyroid should be checked.

Most physicians witness the value of good patient education long before they have completed their formal medical training. It might be said that a girl named Barbara had a lot to do with the beginnings of this book. She arrived one night on the medical service at the Hospital of the University of Pennsylvania when L.C.W. was a young intern. She was seriously ill with uncontrolled diabetes—a condition known as *ketoacidosis.* During that first night of treatment Barbara's understanding of her medical condition was impressive, and the benefits of that understanding were obvious. Her knowledge about diabetes had helped her to *do the right things at home* to control her blood sugar as she began to get sick. It also made her aware of her limitations and told her *when to come to the hospital* as the condition worsened. In the hospital *she was not anxious about her illness* because she knew what to expect as her treatment continued. Instead *she was prepared to participate in her treatment.* She related a clear history of the events leading to her present problem, knew the names and dosages of her medications and the details of her diet, and was familiar with the diabetic complications that she had experienced. Finally, her understanding of her condition *prepared her to learn more about diabetes* while she was in the hospital, knowledge that would help her manage her health better in the future. Barbara had learned about her condition, in part from talking with her physicians. But some of Barbara's understanding of her disease had come from reading *How to Live with Diabetes*, a book written for diabetic patients by Henry Dolger, M.D., and Bernard Seeman.

While practicing together in the Thyroid Unit of the Massachusetts General Hospital, we discovered a mutual interest in patient education and a desire to write a similar book for thyroid patients. As such, it is intended for people who know they have a thyroid problem and who can use it to review and expand upon information given to them by their physicians about their condition. However, we hope this book will reach a wider audience, for many people have thyroid conditions that have not yet been recognized. Unlike diabetes, which usually makes a patient noticeably sick from the start of the illness, thyroid conditions usually begin gradually and may remain unnoticed for months or years. We hope this book will help some of our readers to identify previously unrecognized thyroid problems in themselves or among their relatives and friends and will serve as their guide to proper medical attention and treatment. We hope other readers will simply enjoy it as an introduction to a fascinating part of the remarkable body in which we live.

We greatly appreciate the help of a large number of patients and friends who have made this book possible by their financial support through the Thyroid Clinical Research Fund at the Massachusetts General Hospital. Patients, too, have contributed meaningfully in other ways, for they teach us much about thyroid and related problems by observing their own conditions and relating these observations to us. We especially appreciate those patients who have permitted us to include their pictures to illustrate particular aspects of thyroid disease, as well as those who have written accounts of their personal experiences with thyroid problems. We feel that such accounts, which communicate a sense of the way people *feel* during thyroid illnesses, may have special meaning for others with similar problems.

We are particularly grateful to our colleagues in the thyroid field who have reviewed portions of this book and given us helpful advice pertaining to their areas of expertise. They include Doctors Gerard Burrow, David Becker, Earle Chapman, John Crawford, Delbert Fisher, William Green, Alvin Hayles, Sidney Ingbar, Farahe Maloof, Edward Rose, Paul Walfish, and Robert Volpé. In a similar way we appreciate the help and comments of family members as well as close personal friends, many of whom have thyroid problems or related conditions. They have given us valuable criticism periodically during numerous manuscript revisions.

We would also like to acknowledge the artistic contributions of Linda Hoffman-Kimball and Alex Gray. Linda's creative drawings highlight the text in many special ways, while Alex's medical illustrations clarify many aspects of thyroid anatomy and function.

We appreciate the friendship and good working relationships that we have enjoyed with our publishing staff at Houghton Mifflin and especially with our capable editors, Ruth Hapgood and Lois Randall. We also are indebted to Ruth DiBlasi, Kelly Gritz, Dianna Lynch, and Sharon Melanson for skilled clerical assistance.

PREFACE TO THE THIRD EDITION

We appreciate the continuing interest in this volume of thyroid information, and are especially grateful for the helpful comments of many patients and colleagues since *Your Thy-*

roid was first published in 1982. This new edition has been extensively revised and expanded to reflect important new understandings of thyroid problems. These advances reflect the high quality of thyroid research being carried out throughout the world.

We have added information about the new sensitive TSH test for diagnosing hypo- or hyperthyroidism, and expanded our chapter on thyroiditis to include new information about thyroid dysfunction after pregnancy. We also have a new section examining the risks posed by radioactive-iodine release from nuclear-reactor accidents and an expanded chapter on thyroid nodules and the increasing use of fine-needle biopsy to ascertain whether cancer is present.

The worldwide problem of iodine deficiency is covered. Though iodine deficiency does not exist in this country, it affects one billion people globally and is the most important thyroid problem in the world today. We believe our readers will want to understand what is now the world's leading cause of preventable mental deficiency. In addition we have expanded our chapters on thyroid-related disorders and drugs that can affect thyroid function, and added new chapters on thyroid problems in older individuals, autoimmunity, and current trends in thyroid research.

Throughout the revised text we have added data on the costs and relative importance of laboratory tests and treatments. Our readers must understand these factors that every physician must consider in the course of diagnosis and treatment of thyroid problems. In addition, in a special appendix, we have provided a summary of the costs of all important thyroid tests and treatments reached by averaging the costs in the three hospitals in which the authors now practice.

Our thanks to our agent, Connie Clausen, our editors Ruth Hapgood, Jeff Doctoroff, and Cathy Repetti and to the supportive staff at Ballantine Books. We welcome back Linda Hoffman-Kimball, whose new illustrations have again helped clarify many points in the text. We especially appreciate the guidance of Dr. Kurt Bloch, Chief of Immunology and Allergy at Massachusetts General Hospital, for his comments and suggestions with the text and illustrations for our new chapter about autoimmunity. Finally, we want to express our appreciation to the many patients, physicians, and interested readers who have written to us with helpful criticism and suggestions. Please keep writing and accept our thanks for your important role in developing this new effort to keep you informed and up-to-date about thyroid problems.

D.S.C., E.C.R., L.C.W.

CHAPTER ONE

General Information: *Normal and Abnormal Thyroid Function, Thyroid Diseases, Thyroid Tests, and Thyroid Treatments*

Your thyroid is one of the many glands in your body that make special chemicals known as hormones. Hormones travel in your bloodstream throughout your body to affect many different parts of your system, including your brain, heart, liver, kidneys, muscles, bones, and skin. Therefore it is not surprising that a change in any hormone level can produce abnormalities all over your body. Once they arrive at a particular tissue, hormones interact with receptors, located either on the outside of the cell or inside the cell in the cytoplasm or nucleus, to trigger a certain function. The particular hormone made by your thyroid gland acts on receptors located in the nucleus, affecting the rate at which many bodily processes happen.

Normally your blood level of thyroid hormone is constant, with little day-to-day variation. However, if the gland becomes diseased, it may produce high thyroid-hormone levels that may speed up body processes, causing symptoms such as rapid heartbeat (palpitations), nervousness, frequent bowel movements, and weight loss as you burn up calories more rapidly. In contrast, a slowly functioning gland may produce less than a normal amount of thyroid hormone, which may slow your heartbeat and make you tired, depressed, and constipated. A low thyroid-hormone level may also cause your skin, hair, and fingernails to grow more slowly, so that they become rough, dry, and brittle. You may gain excess weight, though you are unlikely to become obese. In short, if your thyroid is underactive, you will probably feel generally "run-down."

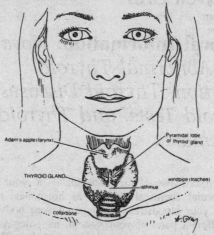

Adam's apple (larynx)

Pyramidal lobe of thyroid gland

THYROID GLAND

windpipe (trachea)

isthmus

collarbone

Figure 1 Your thyroid gland is normally located in the front of your neck below your Adam's apple.

Your thyroid is normally found in the front of your neck (Figure 1). Its two halves, or lobes, normally weigh about one ounce. They lie on either side of your windpipe, just below your "Adam's apple," and are joined together by a narrow band of thyroid tissue known as the *isthmus*. Occa-

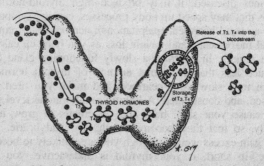

iodine

Release of T3, T4 into the bloodstream

THYROID HORMONES

Storage of T3, T4

T3

T4

Figure 2 Manufacture, storage, and release of thyroid hormones.

sionally a small amount of thyroid tissue will project upward from the isthmus along your windpipe. This tissue, called the *pyramidal lobe*, is a reminder that, before you were born, your thyroid migrated from its place of origin at the back of your tongue down to the front of your neck.

HOW THE THYROID WORKS

Thyroid-hormone production starts with iodine. Iodine is found in many foods, especially seafood, salt, bread, and milk. The thyroid takes this dietary iodine from your bloodstream and uses it to make thyroid hormones (Figure 2). The two most important of these hormones are *triiodothyronine (T3)* and *thyroxine (T4)*. (The nicknames *T3* and *T4* refer to the number of iodine atoms contained in each hormone molecule: There are three iodine atoms in T3 and four in T4.) These hormones are stored within your thyroid. When they are needed, they are released into your bloodstream and transported throughout your body attached to special carrier proteins. After entering the cells of your body tissues they go into nuclei at the center of each cell, where they attach to specific receptors (Figure 3).

Although your thyroid has some inherent ability to produce thyroid hormone by itself, its function is governed largely by the pituitary gland, located at the base of your brain. When your level of thyroid hormone falls too low, the pituitary responds by producing thyroid-stimulating hormone (TSH). If your thyroid is healthy, it responds to TSH by working harder, thereby raising the blood level of thyroid hormone back to normal.

Several factors seem to influence the way the pituitary gland controls thyroid function. A low blood level of thyroid hormone, for example, appears to influence the pituitary gland directly, provoking an increase in TSH release. On the other hand the pituitary is itself under the control of still-higher centers in the brain, including the *hypothalamus* and the cerebral cortex (Figure 3). The interactions between these higher centers of the brain and the thyroid are currently under careful study by research workers.

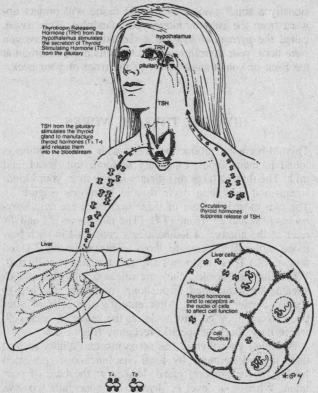

Thyrotropin Releasing
Hormone (TRH) from the
hypothalamus stimulates
the secretion of Thyroid
Stimulating Hormone (TSH)
from the pituitary

hypothalamus

TRH

pituitary

TSH

TSH from the pituitary
stimulates the thyroid
gland to manufacture
thyroid hormones (T₃, T₄)
and release them
into the bloodstream

Circulating
thyroid hormones
suppress release of TSH.

Liver

Liver cells

Thyroid hormones
bind to receptors in
the nuclei of cells
to affect cell function

cell
nucleus

T₄   T₃

Figure 3   The Hypothalamic-Pituitary-Thyroid Axis.

FACTORS INVOLVED IN THYROID DISEASES

Many things can go wrong with your thyroid gland: It can
produce too much hormone (hyperthyroidism) or too little
(hypothyroidism); it can become infected or inflamed (thyroiditis); it can develop a cyst or a tumor. Perhaps the most
common thyroid abnormality is a *goiter*, a simple enlarge-

ment of the thyroid gland. More than one of these conditions may exist or develop over time in a single patient, and different but related thyroid abnormalities may occur in several members of the same family. Although researchers still do not understand all of the mechanisms that produce thyroid disease, we do know a lot about some of the factors involved.

Genetics

The tendency to develop some thyroid problems appears to be inherited. The best studied of these conditions are some rare disorders that result from a failure in the production of thyroid hormone. In some of these disorders the thyroid has difficulty getting enough iodine from the bloodstream. In others there is a problem with the use of the iodine to make the more complex thyroid-hormone molecules.

Heredity also appears to have a role in most instances in which the thyroid changes its level of function and becomes either overactive or underactive. Yet even those who have inherited the tendency to develop one of these thyroid conditions may never become ill. Therefore thyroid disease within a family may seem to "skip" generations. You may have a thyroid problem and, though your parents seem healthy, you may learn of a grandparent who had thyroid trouble too. In other instances several different thyroid problems will show up in one family. Some relatives may develop overactive thyroids, and others may develop underactive thyroids; some may become very sick, while others may be only mildly affected.

Sex

Virtually all thyroid disorders appear to be more common in women than in men. Hyperthyroidism, for example, is four to eight times more likely to occur in women than in men. As of now we don't know why women have this unusual tendency. Nevertheless this should be a future research priority for those of us interested in women's health issues.

Age

If your thyroid is going to become overactive, you will probably be somewhere between the ages of twenty and forty when it happens. On the other hand if your thyroid fails, it will be more likely to do so at a much later age—usually after you reach fifty. Similarly certain types of thyroid tumors tend to occur in young people, while others are more common in older individuals. Unfortunately the reasons for these interesting age differences remain completely obscure.

Diet

Despite the efforts of many health organizations, there are millions of people in the world (especially in remote mountainous areas) who do not get enough iodine in their diets. As a result they have an increased tendency to develop goiters and serious hypothyroidism. In America, on the other hand, iodine deficiency does not exist. Our problem is the opposite: our diets contain a more-than-adequate supply of iodine, and we may get even more in medicines, health foods, or dyes that are used to X-ray our kidneys, gall bladder, or spinal canal. Too much iodine can abruptly raise or lower thyroid activity in some people with underlying thyroid disease. Fortunately most of us are unaffected when we are exposed to excessive amounts of iodine. (See Chapter 15 for further information about this public health problem.)

Some foods contain goitrogens, chemicals that can cause goiter by interfering with thyroid-hormone production. Such foods include cabbage, kale, rutabaga, and turnips. However, the amount of goitrogen in these foods is so low that it would take vast quantities of one or more of them to cause a significant change in thyroid function. Soybean extracts are also capable of producing thyroid enlargement by decreasing the amount of iodine that is absorbed from the intestine. In the 1950s, for example, soy protein was found to be the cause of goiter and iodine deficiency in infants who were fed soy formula instead of milk because of milk allergy. This problem was corrected simply by adding some iodine to the soy formula. Soy protein is now being used in increasing quantities in adult foods as an inexpensive source of protein. At present there is no evidence that it is doing us any harm, probably because of the abundance of iodine in our diets.

Medication

Sometimes a medication will change thyroid function. For example, lithium, a drug used to treat certain psychiatric disorders, can cause both goiter and hypothyroidism in some people. Governmental agencies carefully test new drugs for side effects, and if you are given a drug that can harm your thyroid, you will probably be warned about it by your physician or pharmacist. You should always read the labels on your medicine bottles.

Radiation

You are being exposed continuously to small amounts of environmental radiation. There is no evidence that the amount of radiation that your thyroid receives in this manner is harmful. On the other hand, if you have a tumor or other medical condition near your thyroid gland that must be treated with a larger dose of X rays, or if your thyroid is exposed to a relatively large amount of environmental radiation (as it might be in a nuclear accident or explosion), it may be seriously affected. Your thyroid may become underactive, but this problem can be corrected if you take thyroid-hormone tablets. The greater concern about radiation exposure is that thyroid cancer could develop. We now know that people who are given radiation treatments to the thyroid area have an increased risk for developing thyroid nodules in the years that follow. Some of these nodules may contain thyroid cancer (see Chapter 12). Finally, a number of patients seem to have developed an overactive thyroid (Graves' disease) following radiation treatments that involved the region of the neck where the thyroid gland is located.

Stress

Stress represents an additional environmental problem, but one that is hard to evaluate. Most physicians who see a lot of patients with thyroid dysfunction are impressed by the fact that the commonest form of hyperthyroidism often follows a period of life stress, such as a death in the family or the loss of a job. Some recent studies suggest that stress can alter the immune system, which in turn may cause changes in thyroid function. In spite of these apparent associations, we still do not know exactly how stress influences your thyroid, or why such stressful situations appear to affect the thyroids of some people more than others. Recently smoking has also been linked to the development of hyperthyroidism, but again, the way in which the disease is triggered by tobacco is unknown.

Infections

Bacterial infections of the thyroid are very rare. Infections due to viruses (such as those that produce the common cold) are more likely to cause thyroid disease and are thought to do so in a disorder called *subacute thyroiditis.*

THYROID TESTS

Highly sensitive and specific methods are now available to measure the blood levels of the thyroid hormones thyroxine (T4) and triiodothyronine (T3), as well as the concentration of the pituitary hormone, thyroid-stimulating hormone (TSH). These tests have almost entirely supplanted the previously used but less precise tests of basal metabolic rate and protein-bound iodine. Measurements of T4 and TSH are the most important tests that physicians perform today to determine the function of the thyroid gland.

Other thyroid blood tests are used to evaluate a phenomenon known as protein binding of thyroid hormone. Some thyroid hormone travels in your blood stream in a "free" or active form, but most (greater than 99 percent) is in a "bound" or inactive form that is held by a chemical attraction to certain proteins in your blood. Only the free form of the hormone can act within your body cells. Factors such as pregnancy or medications may alter the amount of bound hormone, but the free level remains normal, so you feel well. In order to estimate the amount of free active hormone, a blood test called the T3 resin uptake or Thyroid Hormone Binding Index (THBI) is used. These are inexpensive, indirect methods of estimating the proportions of active and inactive hormone. When more precise information is required, it is also possible to measure your blood level of free thyroid hormone, as well as the concentrations of the thyroid-binding proteins themselves. The most important of all these thyroid-function blood tests is the measurement of TSH. Fortunately new technologies have made this measurement both highly specific and sensitive. If you suspect you have an abnormality in thyroid-gland function, the TSH measurement can either confirm or refute this possibility with great reliability.

One of the most important advances in thyroid research came in the late 1930s, when physicians learned how to use radioactive iodine to study thyroid function. Since the thyroid gland uses iodine to make thyroid hormone, physicians can use radioactive iodine in several ways to diagnose and treat thyroid problems. If you have a radioactive-iodine uptake test, you will be given a tiny amount of radioactive iodine, usually contained in a small capsule that is easily swallowed. The radioactive iodine (or *radioiodine*) is concentrated in your thyroid gland. Twenty-four hours later a radiation detector or counter held in front of your thyroid gland tells your physician the exact percentage of radioiodine that has been taken up by your thyroid. If your thyroid is overactive, it may take up nearly all of the iodine you swallowed, but if it is underactive, it will usually take up very little. If your thyroid is inflamed (thyroiditis), it may also take up very little iodine.

You may be found to have low radioiodine uptake if you are taking thyroid-hormone tablets or if you have ingested excessive amounts of iodine in medicine or food (such as certain cough remedies, vitamins, and kelp). Similarly a low radioiodine uptake will occur in the weeks following the administration of iodine-containing dyes that have been used to X-ray your kidneys, gall bladder, or other organs. Under these circumstances the test would not accurately reflect the activity of your thyroid.

Your doctor may also want to do a thyroid scan. Here the radiation detector in front of your neck is attached to a scanner, which can draw pictures showing the pattern of radioiodine within your thyroid gland. The procedure takes just a few minutes and is done while you are lying comfortably on an examining table. Thyroid scans may also be performed with another radioactive material known as *technetium.* Technetium is less expensive and faster than radioiodine. The scan can be done twenty minutes after technetium is taken.

A thyroid scan may provide valuable information in a variety of situations. If your thyroid gland is overactive, the scan indicates whether the entire gland is abnormal or just parts of it are overactive (such areas are sometimes referred to as "hot nodules" because of their excessive activity and the picture they make in a thyroid scan). Unfortunately a scan is not very helpful in evaluating thyroid lumps that are suspected of containing cancer. Thyroid cysts, harmless tumors, and cancers all tend to concentrate radioiodine poorly. On the other hand if a lump within the thyroid shows a normal or increased uptake of radioiodine in the thyroid scan, that is a strong indication that the lump does not contain cancer. (Figures 4–8 are different thyroid-scans.)

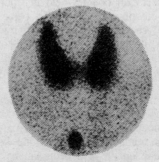

Figure 4   A normal thyroid scan.

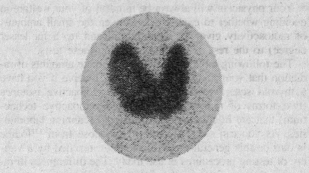

Figure 5 An inactive or "cold" nodule.

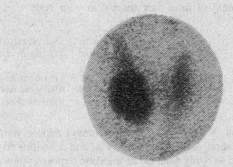

Figure 6 An overactive or "hot" nodule.

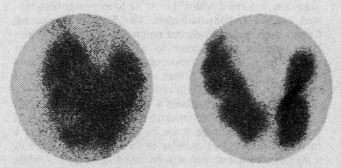

Figure 7 & 8 Multinodular goiters show several areas of increased and decreased activity.

Your physician will always be mindful of your welfare in deciding whether to expose you to even the small amounts of radioactivity given to your thyroid and (to a far lesser degree) to the rest of your body during these tests.

The following table gives the approximate amounts of radiation that your thyroid and your body receive if you have a thyroid scan. We include all three radioactive isotopes (two forms of radioactive iodine and radioactive technetium) that are in common use in thyroid scanning laboratories. As you can see, only the thyroid dose from ^{131}Iodine is outside this general range of radiation reached by a variety of testing procedures in use today. The differences in radiation dosage given by the different isotopes depend upon the amounts of energy that they deliver to body tissues as well as the length of time they remain in your body.

Radiosiotope	Usual Scan Dose	Radiation Delivered to Thyroid	Whole body
^{131}Iodine	30–60 microcuries	33–66 rads	0.014–0.028 rads
^{123}Iodine	100–400 microcuries	1.1–4.4 rads	0.003–0.012 rads
^{99m}Technetium	5,000–10,000 microcuries	1–2 rads	0.06–0.12 rads

For comparison, X rays made of your kidneys expose your body to a radiation dose of about 2 rads, and a barium enema performed to x-ray your large intestine exposes you to slightly more radiation. Today almost all routine thyroid scans are performed with ^{123}I or ^{99m}Te to minimize both thyroid and whole-body radiation. The Nuclear Regulatory Commission recommends that no one exceed 5 rads whole-body radiation in one year, so we are within that "safe range." Even so, your physician will perform such tests only if the radiation exposure is justified by the potential value of the information so obtained.

If more information about a thyroid nodule is needed, your physician may recommend a second type of thyroid picture, one that can be made by using sound waves in a manner similar to that of radar. In this procedure, known as a *thyroid ultrasound*, you will be asked to lie quietly while a small instrument known as a *transducer* sends sound waves through your thyroid gland. The sound waves passing through the tissue echo back to the transducer and produce a picture of your thyroid gland. Dark spaces appear where cysts are found, while solid tumors show as a different pattern of light-and-dark markings.

There are also occasions in which your physician may want to obtain a small sample of your thyroid tissue in order to find out whether a nodule contains thyroid cancer or to understand why your gland has enlarged. In some instances a *fine needle aspiration biopsy* of the thyroid can be done. In this test, after numbing the skin of your neck with a local anesthetic, the physician penetrates the thyroid with a small needle through which a tiny amount of tissue can be removed for examination under a microscope. If the tissue contains cancer, removal of the nodule is necessary. Needless to say, the finding of a thyroid cyst or other harmless lump by means of a thyroid biopsy has saved many thousands of patients from unnecessary thyroid surgery. (See the discussion of a thyroid biopsy in chapter 10.)

A variety of other tests can be used to understand specific thyroid problems. Some of these involve injections of hormones that stimulate your thyroid or pituitary gland in order to find out more about how your thyroid is working. Such tests can be particularly helpful when thyroid disease is suspected, but the more conventional tests have failed to pinpoint the problem. These procedures will be described later in this book when we discuss their use in the evaluation of specific thyroid diseases.

THYROID TREATMENTS

If your thyroid is overactive and producing too much thyroid hormone, it can be controlled in three ways: medication (pills), thyroid surgery, and radioactive iodine. Some medications interrupt the manufacture of thyroid hormones, while others work by blocking the action of the hormones on body tissues. Your thyroid blood level will be reduced, of course, if a surgeon removes part of your thyroid gland, since that is where the hormone is coming from. Radioactive iodine can also be used to treat overactivity of the thyroid gland, since radiation will damage thyroid tissue and decrease hormone production. The amount of radioactive iodine needed to damage thyroid tissue and thus treat hyperthyroidism is much larger than the amount used in a thyroid scan. Furthermore, we use 131-I, which causes more radiation effect on thyroid tissue than the less-damaging 123-I usually used in scans.

If your thyroid is underactive, thyroid-hormone supplements can be given in tablet form to raise your thyroid blood level to normal. These hormones may be helpful in reducing the size of nodules or large goiters in some patients.

Thyroid cancers are best treated by surgery aimed at removing all of the cancer. The use of radioactive iodine can also be helpful, particularly if the tumor is too widespread to be removed surgically. Finally, thyroid-hormone medicine is always used to reduce the spread of a thyroid cancer that cannot be removed entirely or to prevent recurrence of a cancer that has been removed.

SUMMARY

We understand what your thyroid gland does, we can accurately and safely test it, and we can almost always tell whether you have thyroid disease and whether it is mild or serious. Drugs, radioactive iodine, and surgery are available to treat thyroid disorders, and often more than one treatment can be used for the same condition. Thus, appropriate treatment can be "tailor-made" for you no matter what sort of thyroid problem you might develop.

CHAPTER TWO

Goiter: *The Big Thyroid*

I've grown a goitre while living in this den, as cast from stagnant streams in Lombardy, or in what other land they hap to be.

—From a sonnet written by Michelangelo
while he was painting the Sistine Chapel

The word *goiter* often frightens patients, who think it means thyroid cancer. Actually the word merely means an enlarged thyroid gland (Figure 9). There are a great many causes of goiter, and ironically cancer is the least common of all.

The Chinese apparently noticed goiters around 1600 B.C. and were even aware that burned sponge and seaweed sometimes made them smaller. Although iodine was not discovered until 1812, we now suspect that it was iodine in the sponge and seaweed that made the Chinese goiters smaller, and that the thyroid glands had enlarged in the first place due to an insufficiency of iodine in the diet. To the ancient Romans, when the neck of a newly married girl swelled, it was taken as a sign that she was pregnant. In some tribal cultures pregnancy was diagnosed when a goiter developed and broke a thread necklace. Michelangelo, like others of his time, thought that goiter appeared after drinking water that contained something that made the neck swell. Instead, as in all of the other examples mentioned, his goiter was probably due to iodine deficiency in the region in which he was living.

For centuries physicians used the term *goiter* to describe almost any kind of throat swelling, not just enlargement of the thyroid. (Indeed the word may have come from the Latin word *guttur*, which means "throat.") This confused their efforts to find the causes and cures for goiter, since they applied the term to so many different conditions.

Nowadays we know that iodine deficiency is the most

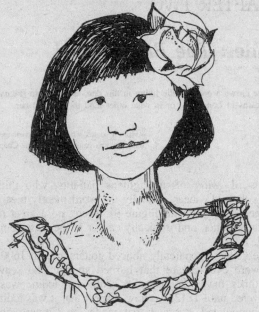

Figure 9 Goiter

common cause of goiter worldwide—in fact it has been estimated that over 500 million people, living mostly in developing countries, suffer from a lack of this essential
nutrient. In some areas of the world simple iodine deficiency is complicated by substances in the diet known as
goitrogens. These agents interfere with the thyroid gland's
ability to use the meager amounts of iodine that *are* available. One common goitrogen is *thiocyanate*, which is found
in root vegetables such as cassava. These roots often consti-
tute a large part of the diet of people in developing countries, especially in Africa. In other parts of the world,
pollutants in the water are believed to contribute to goiter
by interfering with normal thyroid function. For example,
natural water contaminants from coal and shale can cause
goiter, in the absence of iodine deficiency, in children living

in southeastern Kentucky. Some medications can also cause goiter; *lithium*, a commonly used psychiatric drug, causes goiter in up to 10 percent of patients who take it.

At one time the area around the Great Lakes was known as the goiter belt because of the high frequency of iodine-deficiency goiter among the people who lived there. Fortunately, due to iodized salt and other iodine-containing foods, this problem no longer exists in America and is rare in other developed countries. If you have a goiter and you live in the United States, the goiter is not due to iodine deficiency in your diet. Rather your thyroid enlargement means that something else is wrong with your thyroid gland.

A physician can only diagnose a goiter if the thyroid is enlarged compared with a "normal-sized" thyroid gland. There are several ways of telling whether the thyroid is enlarged. The relatively crude standard used by the World Health Organization is that each lobe of your thyroid gland should be no larger than your thumb. As a general rule, if your thyroid is visible, it is enlarged. The most sensitive way of detecting thyroid enlargement is with a technique that employs sound waves called *ultrasound*. Using ultrasound, researchers have determined that the thyroid in an adult should be no larger than approximately 20 cubic centimeters, the equivalent of about 2 teaspoons for each lobe.

The presence of a goiter may mean that your thyroid is becoming overactive. If so, you may also have other evidence of hyperthyroidism, such as a rapid pulse, nervousness, weight loss, diarrhea, and shaky hands. On the other hand a goiter may be the first sign that your thyroid is failing. In that case falling blood levels of thyroid hormone have caused your pituitary gland, located at the base of your brain, to release thyroid-stimulating hormone (TSH), which has caused your thyroid to grow larger. If this is your problem, you may also have other complaints of hypothyroidism, including fatigue, mental dullness, constipation, and a dislike for cold weather. Often thyroid failure and goiter will be due to an inflammation of your thyroid gland known as *chronic lymphocytic thyroiditis*. Such an inflammation is not apparently associated with an infection. Yet, like arthritis or bursitis, the reaction can cause damage to body tissues like the thyroid. At other times goiter and thyroid failure may happen because of treatment your physician may have given you in the past to control an overactive thyroid.

Rarely a goiter will appear due to an inherited condition that is causing your thyroid to function ineffectively. Your thyroid may be unable to collect iodine from your bloodstream in a normal way, or there may be some other problem in the manufacture of thyroid hormone within your thyroid gland. These so-called *metabolic abnormalities* are rare, but it can be helpful to you and your relatives to identify their presence within your family.

A goiter may also develop in association with an infection of your thyroid gland. If so, your thyroid will probably be very painful, and there may be other evidence of the infection, including fever, chills, sluggishness, and aching muscles.

Sometimes what seems to be a generalized enlargement of your entire thyroid gland will prove instead to be a lump or *nodule* that has appeared within the gland. Fortunately most of these nodules do not contain cancer but are due instead to benign (harmless) tumors, fluid-filled *cysts*, or other harmless conditions.

Finally, and *most common of all*, you may develop a goiter without any change in the activity of your thyroid, without inflammation or infection, and without evidence of a cyst or tumor. This type of thyroid enlargement has several names. Some physicians probably use the term *simple goiter* because it rarely causes complications. Others refer to it as *nontoxic goiter* because it usually doesn't make you sick. We prefer to call such conditions *multinodular goiters* because they all contain many small nodules and tend to become more obviously lumpy in later years. Such goiters tend to run in families and, like most thyroid problems, are more common in women than in men. They usually function normally, but may cause hyperthyroidism, especially in elderly patients.

If you develop a goiter, you should have a thyroid evaluation, including an examination by a physician and tests of thyroid functions. This is important, because your goiter may be the first sign of a thyroid problem, and prompt evaluation and early treatment may keep you from becoming seriously sick.

During your examination your physician will ask you about symptoms that might indicate a change in the function of your thyroid gland, and about other symptoms suggestive of compression of nearby structures in the neck, such as neck discomfort, difficulty swallowing or breathing, or hoarseness. He or she will also want to know whether other members of your family have had thyroid problems, for your goiter may be the first indication that you have a similar condition.

The thyroid tests that your physician chooses to help find the cause of your goiter will depend in part on what has been found during your examination. If your physician suspects an overactive or underactive thyroid, tests that measure your blood level of thyroid hormone and pituitary hormone TSH may be helpful. Blood tests may also reveal the presence of substances known as *autoantibodies* in your blood—evidence that your thyroid is affected by autoimmune thyroiditis. *Radioactive scans* can help by showing the function of your entire thyroid or of nodules within your thyroid gland. An ultrasound thyroid picture made with sound waves can also be helpful in distinguishing between a solid thyroid nodule and a fluid-filled cyst. Finally, it is even possible that your physician will obtain cells from your thyroid gland tissue to examine under a microscope. That procedure, known as a thyroid needle biopsy, can be especially helpful if cancer is suspected.

Since most goiters seem to work perfectly well and do not contain cancer, your physician may decide that no treatment is necessary unless your thyroid grows so big that it becomes unsightly or causes hoarseness, difficulty in swallowing, or discomfort in your neck. In such cases you may be given thyroid hormone tablets to suppress the function of your pituitary gland, which normally controls your thyroid.* By inhibiting the release of thyroid-stimulating hor-

---

*Several recent studies have suggested that thyroid-hormone-suppression therapy of thyroid nodules may not work any better than a placebo (Gharib H et al. *New England Journal of Medicine* 1987; 317: 1–8. Reverter JL et al. *Clinical Endocrinology* 1992; 36: 25–28. Nevertheless

mone (TSH) from your pituitary gland, the thyroid tablets may cause your goiter to decrease in size and thereby relieve your discomfort. If the goiter does not shrink with hormone treatment, it can be removed surgically, although an operation is rarely necessary. On the other hand if tests reveal that a problem such as a medication, a change in thyroid function, or a cancer has caused your goiter, your physician will treat you for that specific problem.

SUMMARY

If your thyroid enlarges, it is probably a harmless multinodular goiter, but it may mean that something else is wrong for which you may need treatment. Therefore you should arrange to have a medical examination and appropriate tests performed by your physician. In the following chapters we will describe in detail many of the problems that can cause goiter and abnormal thyroid function, which may be disclosed by your medical examination.

---

many clinicians believe that some patients will respond to thyroid-hormone therapy, and still use it in most patients with benign thyroid nodules, at least for six to twelve months. A recent study supports this idea: La Rosa GL, et al. Levothyroxine and potassium iodide are both effective in treating benign solitary cold nodules of the thyroid. *Annals of Internal Medicine* 122 (1995) 1–8.

CHAPTER THREE

A Patient's Guide to Autoimmunity

> Although lymphocytes have been studied for over a hundred years, not a single function can yet be ascribed to them with any confidence, and their role in the body remains both an enigma and a challenge.

> —From Towell, O.A. The Lymphocyte.
> *International Review of Cytology.* 1958; 7: 236

Your immune system is essential to your health. It is responsible for protecting you from foreign invaders such as bacteria and viruses and from abnormal cells such as cancer cells. When this system breaks down, as it does in individuals infected by the AIDS virus, the body loses its natural resistance and may ultimately succumb to an overwhelming infection or a tumor.

In this chapter we will present basic information about this incredibly complex system before we describe those thyroid conditions that can develop when your immune system goes awry.

THE NORMAL IMMUNE RESPONSE

Under normal circumstances your immune system recognizes foreign invaders or tumor cells as "nonself" and protects you by promptly attacking and destroying them.

Let's suppose, for example, that a new bacteria that has never infected your body before comes floating down your blood stream. Suddenly its presence is detected by a special sort of watchdog cell known as a *macrophage*. As shown in Figure 10, the macrophage is covered with molecules especially coded by a part of your genetic system known as *MHC* which stands for *major histocompatibility gene com-*

plexes. (We never promised that the terms would be simple in immunology.)

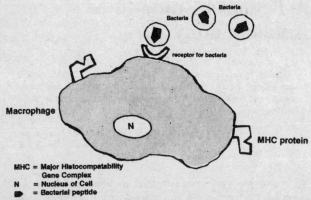

Figure 10   Bacteria is about to attach to macrophage cell receptor.

Something tells these MHC proteins that the new bacteria contains protein foreign to your body, and if the macrophage gets an opportunity, it captures the bacteria and engulfs it, creating a *vacuole* (Figure 11). Inside this container a rise in acidity and enzyme actions break down much of the bacteria, leaving only a critical tiny part known as the *antigen* attached to the MHC protein (Figure 12). The antigen-MHC protein complex then rises to the surface of the cell from which the closely bound bacterial and

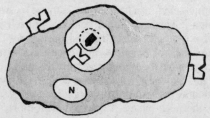

Figure 11   Bacteria and MHC complex in a vacuole within the macrophage.

MHC proteins protrude into the surrounding tissue fluid (Figure 13).

Just about that time a passing white blood cell known as a *helper T lymphocyte* detects the protruding complex. This helper T cell somehow realizes that it has a receptor that neatly fits the exact shape of the MHC-antigen particle and makes the hookup (Figure 14).

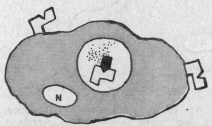

Figure 12 As bacteria is partially destroyed in vacuole, a peptide fragment of one of its proteins becomes attached to the MHC molecule.

This coupling produces a cascade of events as a series of hormones known as *cytokines* are manufactured and released by the involved cells. The T cell releases a cytokine *interferon gamma*, which causes the macrophage, now referred to as the *antigen-presenting cell*, to make other cytokines including *interleukin-1*, or *IL-1*. IL-1 activates the T cells, which in turn make still more cytokines, including *interleukin-2*, which increases the activity and number of T cells. Thus in a very short time, and with great specificity, an army of defenders is raised against the invading bacteria (Figure 15).

Soon other cytokines released by the aroused T cells (*interleukins 4, 5,* and *6*) call out more defenders. These are another type of lymphocyte known as *B cells*. The B cells are the ones that make antibodies—proteins known as *immunoglobulins*—that can attack and destroy the invading bacteria. Some important extra help is offered against the invading bacteria by still another type of lymphocyte known as *killer cells*. These cells can act directly on the bacteria, attaching to them and destroying them.

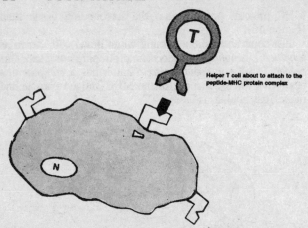

Figure 13 The vacuole recycles to the cell surface, fuses with the surface, then "opens", allowing MHC-peptide complexes to be displayed at cell surface.

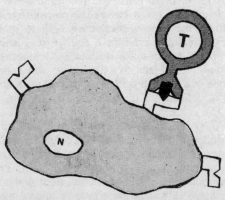

Figure 14 T cell lymphocyte attached to bacterial peptide-MHC protein complex on surface of antigen-presenting cell.

Finally, to create some balance in the overall antibacterial "war effort," at the same time that helper T cells are promoting antibody production by the B cells as described above, other lymphocytes, known as *suppressor T cells*, are quieting down B-cell activity. The result should be a controlled battle, in which the army of invading bacteria is ultimately destroyed.

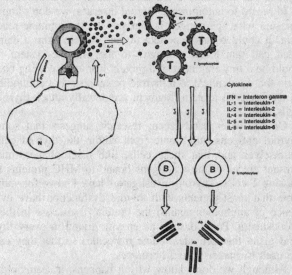

Figure 15   Interactions via cytokines increase T cell number and activity as well as antibody production by B cells.

IMMUNE SYSTEM ERRORS CAUSE AUTOIMMUNE DISEASE

Lest you think the immune system overly complicated, remember that we want a lot of opposition to invading foreign substances, but we only want to destroy the bad ones and not waste time and energy defending against harmless proteins. Above all, we do not want accidentally to destroy our own body tissues, which are proteins too. If we did so in random fashion, we would soon self-destruct.

In reality about 25 percent of individuals do seem to have a problem that results in their having the unfortunate capacity to make antibodies to fragments of some of their own body cells.* If those cells are pancreatic cells, the result is diabetes. If they are thyroid cells, the thyroid may malfunction. Such diseases due to antibody reactions against our own tissues are termed *autoimmune disorders*.

In regard to autoimmune thyroid diseases, we don't know for sure what the antigen is that sets off the immune reaction. It could be an imperfect thyroid protein from a damaged cell that looks "foreign" to the immune system. It could be a tiny fragment of a protein from an invading bacteria that is identical to a thyroid protein, so that antibodies to the bacterial protein fragment accidentally attack thyroid cells, too.

On the other hand recent research suggests that some thyroid antigens may come from within the thyroid cells themselves and that these cells, like macrophages, may present pieces of these antigens bound to MHC proteins to passing T cells. Thyroid investigators have known for some time that most patients with thyroid dysfunction have evidence of antibodies against the protein *peroxidase* in their bloodstream. Peroxidase is an enzyme found in every thyroid gland that activates iodine molecules so that they can be used to make thyroid hormones.

Although we don't know why it happens, it seems clear that individuals who have the capacity to develop thyroid autoimmune problems also have the capacity to make antibodies against peroxidase. Perhaps there is too much of it,

---

*Nearly 17 percent of women manifest a tendency toward autoimmune chronic thyroiditis by developing an increased serum TSH level by the age of sixty. Many other men and women show a tendency to autoimmunity at various ages when they develop such conditions as Graves' disease, insulin-dependent diabetes, pernicious anemia, lupus, Sjögren's syndrome, ileitis, colitis, multiple sclerosis, and rheumatoid arthritis. Because so many people inherit this tendency for autoimmune disorders, scientists are working hard to alter their immune systems so that the self-destructive antibodies that cause these medical problems never appear or are controllable when they do develop.

or perhaps it's being overproduced or made with a slight imperfection. Whatever the case, the thyroid follicular cell itself, the cell in which peroxidase lives and works to help make thyroid hormones, may suddenly decide that peroxidase is a foreign invader, engulf it, and present it to T lymphocytes. The immune reaction that follows results in the production of antibodies against our own thyroid tissues.

Once such antibodies appear, things might not be too bad if their activity was short-lived and balanced by suppressor T cells. But there is evidence that individuals with the inherited tendency to autoimmune thyroid disorders have a problem with their suppressor T cells. Either there are too few of them or they are not active enough to control antithyroid antibody production. Thus the antibodies persist and affect thyroid-cell function in an ongoing manner.

More research must be done before we know which of these or other possible scenarios is really true. Perhaps it's a combination of immune malfunctions, or it may be that different mechanisms produce different disorders. Whatever the true defects prove to be, they result in the appearance of antibodies to our own thyroid tissue, antibodies that stay around and can produce long-term thyroid effects.

ANTITHYROID ANTIBODIES AND THYROID DISEASE

The function of your thyroid gland is normally regulated by *thyroid-stimulating hormone (TSH)*, which is made by the pituitary gland, in your brain. TSH travels to your thyroid via the bloodstream, where it interacts with small protein complexes on thyroid-cell surfaces known as *TSH receptors*. The most important antithyroid antibodies appear to be those that are made against these TSH receptors.

As shown in Figure 16, some of these antibodies stimulate thyroid production of thyroid hormones just like TSH itself. Here the result would be hyperthyroidism. Other antibodies block the receptors, preventing TSH from properly stimulating these cells. If enough TSH receptors are blocked, thyroid function declines, causing hypothyroidism.

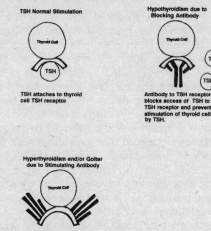

Figure 16   Normal-abnormal states of thyroid receptors.

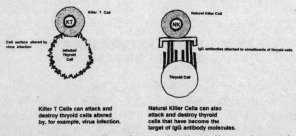

Figure 17   Killer T Cells and Natural Killer Cells can destroy thyroid cells.

A third type of antibodies appears to attach to other receptors on thyroid cells, stimulating tissue growth. Patients with such antibodies may develop thyroid enlargement known as *goiter*. Finally, killer cell lymphocytes can attach to and destroy thyroid cells, producing irreversible hypothyroidism (Figure 17).

In reality of course the immune system is far more complex than described above. Immunology is also one of the most rapidly advancing fields of research in medicine today. When we look back ten years hence and consider updating this book, we may be embarrassed by new discoveries in immunology that will have made this edition quite out of date.

Despite these misgivings, we hope that this chapter explains enough of our current understanding of autoimmunity to set the stage for the following chapters, which describe thyroid disorders caused by immune dysfunction.

CHAPTER FOUR

The Overactive Thyroid:
Hyperthyroidism Caused by Graves' Disease (Diffuse Toxic Goiter)

A lady, aged twenty, became affected with some symptoms which were supposed to be hysterical. . . . After she had been in this nervous state about three months it was observed that her pulse had become singularly rapid. . . . She next complained of weakness on exertion and began to look pale and thin. . . . It was observed that the eyes assumed a singular appearance, for the eyeballs were apparently enlarged. In a few months . . . a tumor, of a horseshoe shape, appeared on the front of the throat and exactly in the situation of the thyroid gland.

—From the clinical lectures delivered by Robert J. Graves, M.D.,
at the Meath Hospital in Dublin, Ireland, during 1834–5
(*London Medical and Surgical Journal*, 1835; 7 pt. 2:516).

The most common type of hyperthyroidism is produced by a generalized overactivity of the entire thyroid gland. This is called *diffuse toxic goiter*—*diffuse* because the *entire* gland is involved in the disease process; *toxic* because the patient appears hot and flushed, as if he or she were "toxic" due to an infection; and *goiter* because the overactivity enlarges the gland. Diffuse toxic goiter is also known as *Graves' disease*, in honor of the Irish physician, Robert J. Graves, who was one of the first to describe this condition and who first noted the protrusion of the eyes that is sometimes associated with it. Between 1 and 2 percent of all people in the United States will develop Graves' disease at some time in their life, and every year about half a million new cases are diagnosed. Graves' disease is three to four times more common in women than in men and typically begins between the ages of twenty and forty.

If you develop Graves' disease, your thyroid will begin to produce more and more thyroid hormone. As it does so, the gland will usually grow larger and will in most cases grow big enough to protrude noticeably at the front of your neck. You may notice the enlargement in your neck yourself, or you may not notice anything until a friend or physician points it out. If the goiter is small, you may only sense the presence of a lump while swallowing. Typically in this form of hyperthyroidism your thyroid gland is not tender, and it is not uncomfortable when you swallow.

As you develop hyperthyroidism, you may lose weight even though you seem to eat plenty of food. You may feel nervous and jumpy and may become quite irritable and quarrelsome. You are likely to perspire more than usual and to dislike hot weather. Your skin may gradually become thin and delicate, and you may notice that you are losing some of the hair on your head. As your fingernails grow more rapidly, you may notice an irregularity of the nail margin, making it difficult for you to keep your fingernails clean. It is also possible that you could develop itchy hives on your skin.

Muscle weakness, especially involving your upper arms and thighs, may make it difficult for you to carry heavy packages or to climb stairs. You may in fact experience such marked leg weakness that you cannot stand up from a squatting position without help. You may notice that your hands shake, and at times this tremor may become so severe that you can't even carry a cup of coffee without its rattling or spilling in its saucer. Your heartbeat may speed up from a normal rate of 70 or 80 to well over 100 beats per minute. Occasionally, without warning, your pulse may quicken, causing very rapid palpitations that last several minutes and then end as mysteriously and abruptly as they began. You are unlikely to have real diarrhea, but your bowel movements may become loose and more frequent.

If you are a woman, your menstrual cycle may change. Your flow may become much lighter, and the interval between menstrual periods may lengthen. More rarely your periods may become irregular or may cease entirely, making it more difficult for you to become pregnant. If pregnancy does occur, there appears to be an increased likelihood that you will have a miscarriage. Women usually notice little change in their breasts, but if you are a man, your breasts may become slightly larger and may be tender.

One of the most puzzling and least understood aspects of Graves' disease is the way it may affect your eyes. Usually the change is simply an elevation of your upper eyelids that makes your eyes appear more prominent (Figure 18). Occasionally, however, swelling of the tissue behind your eyeballs may cause actual protrusion of the eyes, known as *exophthalmos* or *proptosis*. Sometimes your eyes will feel dry or become red and irritated. A few patients have involvement of their eye muscles that may make them see double. In its most extreme (and very rare) form, the nerve to one or both of your eyes becomes inflamed and you may

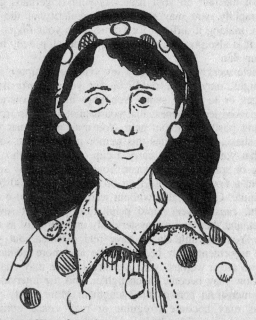

Figure 18 Hyperthyroidism may make your eyes appear larger than normal.

have trouble with your vision. This condition is known as *optic neuropathy.*

Elevation of the upper eyelids may be seen in anyone who has a high level of thyroid hormone, even someone who is taking thyroid hormone tablets in excess. The other things that can happen to your eyes in Graves' disease are unrelated to your blood level of thyroid hormone. If you are one of the people with Graves' disease who develops eye inflammation and protrusion, the eye problems will probably begin when you first become hyperthyroid. Quite often, however, eye problems and thyroid overactivity occur at different times, occasionally separated from one another by many years. Very rarely a person may develop eye trouble as the only manifestation of Graves' disease.

Eye disease is therefore one problem that occurs only in the type of hyperthyroidism that is caused by Graves' disease. Another condition unique to Graves' disease is a very rare skin disorder that appears on the front of your legs and rarely on top of your feet. This is called *pretibial myxedema* and takes the form of a lumpy, reddish-colored thickening of your skin. It is usually painless and not serious. As with the eye trouble in Graves' disease, pretibial myxedema may occur anytime. Its appearance does not necessarily coincide with the beginning of your thyroid problem, nor is its severity related to your blood level of thyroid hormone.

One of the rarest manifestations of Graves' disease is *thyroid acropachy,* which causes the tissues around the base of the nails to become swollen, but not painful. *Periodic paralysis* is yet another condition occasionally seen in patients with Graves' disease. This disorder causes sudden attacks of profound weakness of all the muscles of the body. In susceptible patients, sugar or starchy foods appear to cause a lowering of the blood potassium level, which prevents normal muscle function. For unknown reasons periodic paralysis is most often seen in Asian men with Graves' disease.

WHAT CAUSES GRAVES' DISEASE?

Graves' disease seems to be caused by the interaction of a variety of different factors, including heredity, your body's immune system, your age, sex hormones, and stress. Some sort of genetic predisposition seems to be needed first, and can be thought of as an inherited *tendency* to develop hyperthyroidism. If you have this factor, you may develop Graves' disease at some time during your life, or you may not, but if you lack this genetic factor, you probably cannot develop this disorder.

This type of hyperthyroidism clearly runs in families. If you have Graves' disease, and if sensitive thyroid tests could be carried out on your relatives, they might show mild thyroid abnormalities in one of your parents and one of your grandparents, in some of your aunts, uncles, brothers, and sisters, and possibly in some of your children as well. Fortunately, few of these relatives will ever become sick enough from their thyroid problems to require treatment. However, as we suggest in Chapter 8, some of them should be checked periodically by their family physician.

Studies in identical twins confirm the importance of genetics in Graves' disease and also show the ability of other factors to modify the disease. Usually either both twins will have Graves' disease or neither develops the problem. But since other factors influence the disease process, twins rarely experience the onset of hyperthyroidism at the same time, and the *course* of the disease in the twins may be quite different.

There appear to be many different factors that can trigger Graves' disease in a person who has inherited a tendency to it. Many thyroid specialists believe that *stress* can play a role in starting the hyperthyroidism, for we all have seen patients in whom a stressful situation, such as a death in the family, has preceded the onset of this condition. *Sex hormones* are also important, for the disease is four to eight times more common in women than in men, and not infrequently begins after a hormonal change such as pregnancy. *Age* also seems to have something to do with the onset of Graves' disease, since it is most likely to appear when you are between the ages of twenty and forty. Finally, your body's *immune system* appears to play a role in the production of this disorder. By an unknown mechanism, substances called *autoantibodies* appear in your blood. These autoantibodies bind to the cells in your thyroid gland and stimulate the thyroid to overactivity by mimicking the effects of pituitary thyroid-stimulating hormone (TSH). This causes the thyroid to enlarge and to make more thyroid hormone. Thus instead of being under the control of your pituitary gland, which is the normal situation, your thyroid becomes controlled by these abnormal antibodies in your blood (see Chapter 3). The immune disorder that characterizes Graves' disease usually develops spontaneously, but recent studies have shown that you could be at increased risk for the disease if your thyroid gland was inadvertently damaged by X rays for cancer therapy in the past or if you are taking one of the new immune-altering drugs such as *interferon* and *interleukin*.

In summary a susceptible person develops Graves' disease because of one or more factors that trigger off thyroid overactivity. As thyroid function increases, more thyroid hormones are released into the blood stream, producing the symptoms of hyperthyroidism.

DIAGNOSING GRAVES' DISEASE

If you go to your doctor with symptoms that suggest an overactive thyroid, the diagnosis can usually be confirmed easily and safely. In your examination your doctor will look for a goiter, a rapid pulse, a tremor, and other evidence of hyperthyroidism. If such evidence is found, a sample of your blood can be tested for the level of the thyroid hormone thyroxine (T4). If your T4 level is high, it confirms the presence of hyperthyroidism.

However, under some circumstances an elevated T4 level is not enough evidence to prove that you have an overactive thyroid. This is because thyroid hormones are carried in your blood mainly in an inactive form attached to certain of your blood proteins, so only a very small amount of your thyroid hormone is free and active. Pregnancy, birth control pills, and other nonthyroid factors may increase the total amount of thyroid hormone bound to protein and therefore give a false impression of hyperthyroidism, even though your "free" or active T4 level remains normal. A T3 resin uptake (T3RU) or thyroid hormone binding index (THBI) are blood tests which offer an inexpensive means of clarifying the situation by telling whether your thyroid-hormone-binding protein is normal. Alternatively your physician can measure the *free* T4 level itself in a sample of your blood, though this procedure is more expensive.

Your doctor may also wish to measure the amount of TSH in your blood. In recent years this test has become an increasingly important method of assessing a patient's thyroid situation. In Graves' disease and in most other forms of hyperthyroidism, your thyroid gland overproduces thyroid hormone on its own, overriding the normal pituitary-gland control mechanism. Your pituitary correctly senses that the level of thyroid hormone in your bloodstream is excessive, and it compensates by releasing less TSH. Levels of TSH in your blood then fall until they are low or undetectable. Until quite recently techniques for measuring TSH were not sufficiently reliable to tell whether a patient's blood TSH level was low, or if it was within normal limits. Nowadays most physicians have access to laboratories where so-called "sensitive" TSH assays are available. These new tests can easily tell whether your TSH level is low, suggesting thyroid overactivity, or normal. This single blood test has replaced the far more time-consuming, expensive, and complicated "TRH test" that used to be done in patients whose thyroid function was only marginally elevated, making it difficult to tell whether they were normal or mildly hyperthyroid. The new assays make it possible to detect even the mildest and most subtle forms of thyroid overactivity. In fact doctors can now diagnose *subclinical hyperthyroidism*, in which the blood levels of thyroid hormones are in the high-normal range but the levels of TSH are low. This milder condition is particularly common in patients whose hyperthyroidism is due to one or more overactive thyroid nodules (see Chapter 5).

If more information is needed, your physician will usually order a *radioactive-iodine uptake* test. Determining that your thyroid gland is using a greater-than-normal amount of iodine helps to exclude other causes of hyperthyroidism, such as thyroid inflammation (*thyroiditis*). Often a picture of your thyroid (*thyroid scan*) will be made at the same time in order to find out whether your entire thyroid gland is overactive, as is the case with Graves' disease, or whether just a portion of the gland is hyperfunctioning, as would be the case in a toxic *nodular* goiter (see Chapter 5).

Occasionally your doctor will measure the level of thyroid autoantibodies in your blood. One type of autoantibody is the *antiperoxidose* antibody (previously called the *antimicrosomal* antibody), which is frequently seen in patients with Graves' disease. It may suggest to your physician that your thyroid overactivity is due to Graves' disease and not some other thyroid disorder. Another type of autoantibody is referred to as *thyroid-stimulating immunoglobulin*, or *TSI*. Although it is not necessary to test for TSIs in all patients, it is helpful in certain patients. These include rare patients with eye problems that are similar to thyroid eye disease but whose thyroid blood tests are normal, and pregnant patients with Graves' disease (see Chapter 13).

THE TREATMENT OF GRAVES' DISEASE

Rest and sedation were the only treatment available for hyperthyroidism until 1884, when a patient was cured by having part of the thyroid gland removed surgically. In the early days of surgery, however, patients were often so sick with hyperthyroidism that many died during the operation. It wasn't until the 1920s that we learned to control the severity of hyperthyroidism before the operation by giving patients iodine drops, which slowed down thyroid function. This simple treatment markedly decreased the risk of surgery for patients with Graves' disease. For a while physicians tried to avoid surgery and treat patients with iodine alone, but although this worked temporarily, control of the disease was unpredictable, and many patients suffered a relapse of hyperthyroidism even while continuing to take iodine drops.

Antithyroid drugs, such as *propylthiouracil (PTU)* and *methimazole (Tapazole)*, have been in use since the 1940s and represent one of the three major forms of treatment currently employed to treat the hyperthyroidism of Graves' disease. These drugs act to prevent the thyroid from manufacturing thyroid hormone. Then, as the production of hormone declines, the symptoms of hyperthyroidism gradually subside. If this is the way your overactive thyroid is treated, you will probably begin to feel better within ten days to two weeks, and you will feel almost well in six to eight weeks.

You will probably take the medication for twelve to twenty-four months, after which your physician will probably stop the drug to see if your hyperthyroidism returns. Current studies indicate that you will have about a 30 percent chance of remaining well without medication. You are likely to be one of the fortunate 30 percent if your hyperthyroidism was mild to begin with or if you started treatment within a few months of the beginning of your illness. If you do experience a remission, your physician will still check you periodically after that to be sure that your thyroid does not become overactive again and also to be sure that thyroid failure does not appear in later years.

Though antithyroid drugs provide an excellent treatment for hyperthyroidism, they have certain peculiarities that you should know about if your doctor prescribes them for you. First, because PTV has a short duration of action, if your doctor prescribes PTV, he or she will probably recommend that you take these medications every six to eight hours, at least to begin with. Many people have difficulty remembering the midday doses. Methimazole is preferred by the authors because its longer duration of action allows it to be taken once a day by most patients.

Second, antithyroid drugs cause allergic reactions in about 5 percent of patients who take them. The most common reaction is a skin rash that is usually red and itchy but, in its extreme form, it may have the appearance of generalized hives. Less often the pills may cause fever, joint pains, or liver disease. A far more serious form of antithyroid drug reaction, which happens to about one of every three hundred patients who take the medication, is a decrease in the neutrophil (white blood cell) count, called *agranulocytosis*, which may lower your resistance to infections. Therefore if you are taking one of these drugs and develop a rash, itching, hives, joint pains, or evidence of an infection (such as fever or sore throat), you should stop taking the drug and **immediately** call your physician. If your physician determines that your problem is drug allergy, another form of treatment will be recommended.

If you have any fever or infection while you are taking an antithyroid medication, you *must* have your white blood cell count measured. If the count shows a normal number of neutrophils, your doctor can restart your antithyroid drug even while your infection is being treated. If the neutrophil count is low, your doctor will begin another form of thyroid treatment. Thereafter your physician will watch you and your blood count very carefully until you are healthy again. Some physicians monitor their patients' white blood cell count routinely. Most doctors have not found this to be practical, since this side effect is quite uncommon. Furthermore the drop in the white blood count can occur suddenly, even if it was normal only a few days before. However, a 1991 Japanese study found that monthly checks of the white blood cell count did identify some patients who had developed this problem before they experienced symptoms of a fever or sore throat.* Since early diagnosis is critical, your physician may decide to test your white blood count periodically if you are taking one of these drugs.

Other recent studies suggest that agranulocytosis is more likely to occur in older patients (in whom radioiodine is the preferred treatment anyway) and is more common in patients given propylthiouracil than in those given methimazole, as long as the dose of methimazole does not exceed 30 milligrams per day.

Even if your white blood cell count has been lowered by the drug, your count will probably return to normal within seven to fourteen days after you stop the medication. But if you continue to take one of these drugs in spite of a falling white blood count, there is risk of a serious and possibly fatal outcome. This possible danger *must* be thoroughly understood by all who take the drugs.

If antithyroid drugs have failed to control your hyperthyroidism, or if they are inappropriate for some other reason,

*Tajiri J, Noguchi S, Murakami T, et al. Antithyroid drug-induced agranulocytosis: The usefulness of routine white blood cell monitoring. *Archives of Internal Medicine.* 1990; 150: 621–24.

doctors can limit your thyroid gland's ability to function with either radioactive iodine or surgery.

Radioactive iodine has been used in the treatment of hyperthyroidism for many years. Studies that were begun in 1939 demonstrated the treatment's effectiveness, and long-term follow-up studies from many medical centers have confirmed its safety. Radioactive iodine in this treatment is the same isotope (^{131}I) used in many laboratories to test thyroid function in uptake and scan procedures, but the treatment dose is of course much larger. Radioiodine is successful in controlling hyperthyroidism because it goes into the thyroid gland and remains there long enough to irradiate—and thus destroy—large amounts of thyroid tissue. Then within days it disappears from the body, either eliminated in the urine or transformed by decay into a nonradioactive state. If the dosage is calculated correctly, you should be well in three to six months, and that is usually what happens. If you are given too little radioactive iodine, you will remain hyperthyroid, but less so than before. Surprisingly, with so many factors to consider in choosing a proper treatment dose of radioiodine, about 80 percent of patients have their hyperthyroidism controlled with a single treatment. Moreover, those who are still hyperthyroid can be given one or more additional doses of radioiodine until they become well.

You may wonder why every hyperthyroid patient isn't treated this way. Radioactive iodine is tasteless and easily dispensed, either as a capsule or in a glass of water. It is so readily absorbed that you don't need to fast when you are given the treatment. Furthermore, radioactive iodine is usually well tolerated and painless, though in rare instances patients have complained of a sore throat or mild thyroid tenderness for two or three days. For all of these reasons a 1990 survey of thyroid specialists in the United States showed that the majority preferred to use radioactive iodine to treat the typical patient with Graves' disease.*

The greatest concern that we have about radioactive iodine—and the reason that we are particularly reluctant to

---

*Solomon B, Glinoer D, Lagasse R, and Wastofsky L. Current trends in the management of Graves' disease. *Journal of Clinical Endocrinology and Metabolism.* 1990; 70: 1518–24.

treat small children in this manner—is its potential for harm to the thyroid or other parts of the body from the radiation used in the treatment. As outlined in detail in Chapter 12, there is no question that X rays and other radioactive substances, including radioactive iodine, can cause benign and malignant tumors in human beings who are exposed to large enough quantities. Yet early worries over possible harmful effects in hyperthyroid patients who were treated with radioiodine have not been borne out in the more than fifty years that we have treated patients in this manner. For example, we have not observed any increased risk of leukemia, thyroid cancer, or other tumors in patients treated with radioiodine when compared with similar patients treated with antithyroid drugs or surgery. Additionally there has been no evidence of infertility or birth defects in children born to women following this treatment. On the other hand, ^{131}I treatment should **never** be given to a woman during pregnancy, because of the risk of damage to the thyroid of the unborn child (see Chapter 13). At present therefore our experience leads us to conclude that radioactive iodine is the treatment of choice for hyperthyroidism in most adults. Moreover, it is now being used increasingly in younger patients as well.

The major problem with radioiodine treatment for hyperthyroidism is the subsequent development of hypothyroidism. If you have Graves' disease, your thyroid will probably become underactive at some future time. However, your thyroid will fail sooner after radioiodine than it will after antithyroid-drug or surgical treatment of your overactive thyroid. Long-term follow-up studies of patients with Graves' disease who have been treated with radioactive iodine reveal that within ten years up to 90 percent of patients so treated will have become hypothyroid. Nevertheless late thyroid failure is not necessarily a reason to avoid the use of radioactive iodine to treat this disease, since the immediate necessity is to reduce thyroid-hormone production; this is accomplished easily and safely with radioiodine. Furthermore when the thyroid gland does fail to function, it can be treated safely and easily with hormone tablets taken just once a day.

There has long been controversy among physicians about possible adverse effects of treatment on the eyes of patients with Graves' disease. In 1992 researchers in Sweden detected a worsening of eye problems in some patients after treatment with radioiodine, compared with similar patients who received antithyroid drugs or surgery to combat their hyperthyroidism.* In the majority of patients this deterioration was mild and did not require any special treatment. The issue is still unsettled, since a number of older research studies found that thyroid treatment had no effect on associated thyroid eye problems, no matter which form of treatment patients received. For now it seems prudent to recommend caution when radioiodine is being considered for patients with more severe degrees of eye involvement.

If radioiodine is given, it is important that hypothyroidism be detected and treated early, since there is a possibility that the resulting hypothyroidism may make eye problems worse. There is also evidence that concurrent treatment with steroids, such as cortisone, may prevent any worsening of the eye problem that may result from radioiodine treatment. If you have eye problems, it is important that you discuss these issues with your doctor before radioiodine is administered. Physicians are continuing to search for other factors to explain why some patients experience worsening of their eye disease in the course of treatment of their Graves' disease.

The key to proper treatment of hyperthyroidism with radioiodine is a careful and prolonged follow-up. Unfortunately a lot of older people were treated with radioiodine many years ago and were told they were "cured" by their radioactive-iodine treatment; they were never warned about late thyroid failure because their physicians didn't know it would happen. Therefore it is our recommendation that if you or someone you know had radioiodine treatment years ago, you should schedule a follow-up thyroid evaluation.

If your physician decides to treat your thyroid with radioactive iodine, it will be because the expected benefits from the treatment outweigh the small risk of harmful side effects to your thyroid and the rest of your body from the radioiodine. But when you return home after your treatment,

*Tallstedt L, Lundell G, Tørring O, et al. Occurrence of ophthalmopathy after treatment for Graves' hyperthyroidism. *New England Journal of Medicine* 1992; 326: 1733–38.

the radioactive iodine in your body can affect those around you. Although the risk to them from your radioiodine is small, if you take some simple precautions, you can minimize their exposure to your radioactivity.

Most of the radioactivity will be eliminated from your body in your urine within forty-eight hours, so those two days are the important time for precautions. During that time your radioactivity can affect those around you, their exposure depending upon how long they are with you and how far away they are from you. Thus we advise our patients to minimize the time they are in close contact with others. Since infants and small children are the most sensitive to such radiation, make a special point of avoiding prolonged close contact with them. For example let someone else hold and feed babies while you sit farther away.

Since radioactive iodine is present in the urine, elderly patients who have problems with bladder control must be especially careful in using the bathroom during the first two days after treatment. Since the radioiodine will also be in saliva, we advise our patients to avoid kissing anyone for forty-eight hours. Finally, radioiodine will be present in breast milk, so if you are breast-feeding, you will have to stop nursing until your doctor says it is safe to start again.

When actual measurements have been carried out in patients' homes, it has been found that a treated patient exposes family members to very little radiation. Nevertheless these simple precautions are worth taking to keep that exposure to a minimum. Many hospitals furnish written guidelines detailing the ways in which you can minimize the exposure to others (see Appendix 2).

Your hyperthyroidism can also be cured by means of surgery, in which most of your thyroid gland is removed. Following such a procedure the thyroid tissue that remains in your neck may still be hyperactive, but since the amount of tissue is less, it cannot produce as much thyroid hormone. Thus your thyroid-hormone blood levels will fall and your symptoms of hyperthyroidism will subside.

To prepare you for surgery, your physician will probably control your thyroid function by treating you for a few weeks with an antithyroid drug. Iodine drops are also usually prescribed during the ten days just before surgery so that there will be less bleeding during your operation.

Most surgeons remove about 90 percent of the thyroid gland in order to be sure that enough tissue is removed to cure the patient. Hypothyroidism may occur immediately after surgery, or may develop later, but if it does occur, it can be treated easily with thyroid-hormone tablets. Patients taking thyroid tablets should feel completely well if their dose of thyroid hormone is correct.

If you elect to have surgical treatment, the major concern for you and your doctor should be the choice of the surgeon who will perform your operation. Head and neck surgery requires the skills of an expert, and most large hospitals have certain surgeons who perform most of the thyroid surgery. The choice of the surgeon is important because surgical complications may be serious. The *recurrent laryngeal nerves*, which supply your vocal cords, pass very near to the thyroid (Figure 19). If your surgeon accidentally cuts one of these nerves during the operation, you will be immediately and permanently hoarse. There is also danger of

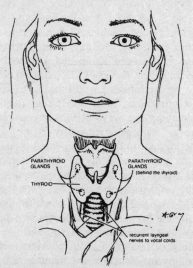

Figure 19 The thyroid and the recurrent laryngeal nerves.

damage to the parathyroid glands, which control your blood calcium level. If that occurs, you may need medication for the rest of your life. Many patients want to know what sort of scar to expect after a thyroid operation. Actually most are invisible within several months. More detailed guidelines to assist you in discussing the choice of a thyroid surgeon with your physician can be found in Appendix 1 at the back of this book.

In summary, if a skilled, experienced thyroid surgeon is not available, radioactive iodine or antithyroid drugs are safer forms of therapy for the hyperthyroidism of Graves' disease. On the other hand if you are allergic to antithyroid drugs or do not want to take radioactive iodine, thyroid surgery can be a very good way to control an overactive thyroid.

No matter which of the three main methods of treatment you and your physician decide upon, your doctor may also prescribe a *beta-adrenergic blocking drug*, such as *atenolol, metoprolol*, or *propranolol*, to block the action of circulating thyroid hormone on your body tissues, slowing your heart rate, lessening nervousness, and generally improving your symptoms within hours. These drugs work so well in hyperthyroidism that, in rare cases, some physicians use them as the sole form of therapy for the disease, but more commonly they are given for temporary relief until thyroid function can be controlled permanently by a more traditional method.

Beta-blocking agents have some disadvantages for a few patients: They may make asthma worse and may decrease the strength of heart-muscle contraction in patients with heart failure. However, since most hyperthyroid patients are young, the latter complication is rarely encountered. Lesser concerns are the drugs' duration of action, which sometimes makes it necessary for patients to take the pills three or four times a day. The authors prefer long-acting drugs of this type to the shorter-acting "parent drug" propanolol (Inderal) because of the more convenient once-a-day dosage. Diabetics should know that these drugs may obscure the warning signs of low blood sugar (hypoglycemia). Finally, beta-blocking agents are not recommended for long-term use in pregnancy or for use near the time of delivery if another treatment is available. In spite of all these potential problems these drugs are usually so safe, they are now in common use in the early stages of treatment of many hyperthyroid patients. They make patients feel better until their thyroid glands can be controlled by other means.

Iodine is another form of therapy. Although iodine alone is not a good treatment for hyperthyroidism, it is often used in conjunction with surgery (noted above) or after radioactive-iodine treatment. During the three to six months while you wait for the radioactive iodine to work, your doctor may prescribe iodine drops or antithyroid drugs to control your hyperthyroidism temporarily. These drugs will be withdrawn gradually as your hyperthyroidism subsides as a result of the radioactive-iodine treatment.

New drugs are constantly under investigation because every treatment has some possible complications. Most patients, however, are easily and safely managed by one of the standard time-tested remedies: antithyroid drugs, radioiodine, or a thyroid operation. But no matter what the therapeutic approach, every patient treated for hyperthyroidism must have at least an annual follow-up examination, including measurements of serum T4 and TSH concentrations, for the rest of his or her life. In this way when hypothyroidism does develop, it will be promptly detected and treated.

Treatment of Graves' Eye Disease

Most patients with Graves' disease never develop a problem with their eyes, or, if they do, it is so mild that no treatment is needed. Often, particularly in the mildest cases, the eye problem simply goes away by itself. More severe eye problems take many forms, but a number of treatments are available. If the main symptoms are eye irritation, tearing, and redness, they can usually be managed with "artificial tears" eyedrops or an eye lubricant ointment. If your lids do not close completely while you are asleep, your doctor may recommend "patching" them closed with paper adhesive tape to prevent damage to your eye from overexposure to the air. Dark glasses may be helpful if bright lights are bothersome, and mild puffiness around the eyes can sometimes be helped by elevating your bed at night or taking a mild diuretic medication. If there are more severe problems with eye swelling, irritation, or protrusion, your physician may recommend additional measures, such as high doses of steroid drugs like cortisone, and X-ray treatments to the back of the eye. The root of these eye problems is an enlargement of the muscles behind the eyes, so these forms of treatment work by reducing the muscle swelling, which lessens the protrusion of the eye and the swelling of surrounding tissues. Occasionally if your eye muscles become swollen and inflamed, you may experience double vision, but special glasses fitted with prisms in the lenses can usually correct mild cases.

Very rarely a patient's eyesight can actually be threatened by Graves' eye disease when swollen eye muscles compress the *optic nerve*, which lies behind the eye and carries visual images to the brain. In this situation steroids, radiation, and eye muscle surgery may all be needed. The surgical procedure, called *orbital decompression*, usually helps. Once the space in the back of the eye is enlarged, the swollen muscles can expand into a new space created by the surgeon in the floor or wall of the orbit. This in turn relieves the pressure behind the eye and permits the eyeball to move back into its normal position inside the orbit. Luckily this kind of treatment is hardly ever needed, but when it is, you should see an eye specialist who is highly experienced in the management of Graves' eye disease.

New research suggests that cigarette smokers are at greater risk for these troubles than non-smokers, so if you smoke and have just developed Graves' disease, stop smoking at once.

SUMMARY

If you have Graves' disease, your overactive thyroid will probably slow down someday and become underactive. This will happen earlier if the treatment used to control your hyperthyroidism is radioiodine or surgery (both of which damage your thyroid) than if your treatment is with antithyroid drugs alone. It might happen, though perhaps not for many years, if you are not treated at all. In short the natural history of Graves' disease appears to be a slow but progressive decline in thyroid function in later years that can be hastened by antithyroid treatment that damages your thyroid gland.

GRAVES' DISEASE

by L. H.

I am twenty-seven years old, and I have had Graves' disease for the past year. In June 1973 I started having vague symptoms that my husband and I overlooked as normal. The only problem that bothered me was the constant sensation of having sand in my eyes. Then, practically overnight, they became inflamed, swollen, and itchy. I immediately went to an eye doctor, who diagnosed a viral infection. But during the rest of the summer my eyes continued to fluctuate between being normal or being symptomatic. I never once thought the other things that were happening to me could be related, so I never mentioned them to the eye doctor who saw me.

I have always been extremely conscious of my weight, so when I found that I had lost fifteen pounds over the course of the summer, I thought it was so terrific, I didn't even question it. I suddenly could eat anything I wanted, in any quantity, and I wouldn't gain any weight.

I work on a ward in a hospital and it is not air-conditioned. Thus my intolerance to heat seemed natural. Everyone complained of the heat, but I seemed to feel it more and to sweat more than anyone else.

Weight loss and heat intolerance were the only two symptoms I had during the first few months of my disease. At the end of the summer, however, everything seemed to reach a peak almost overnight. I knew something was very wrong when my eyes became prominent and my lids retracted to the point where I could not close my eyes easily. I couldn't sleep well at night. I was very jumpy and irritable with people around me. After doing the mildest form of exercise my legs would feel like rubber and start shaking. I kept having bouts of diarrhea, and my heart felt it was pounding very hard.

My overactive thyroid was discovered by my doctor at the end of the summer, and suddenly all of these symptoms made sense. I wasn't sick because my husband or anyone else was trying to provoke me and irritate me; it was me all along. Unfortunately my being so jumpy and excitable at this time made it very hard for me to accept my disease. I felt as if I was constantly wound up, and the slightest provocation would cause me to explode. It's a terrible feeling to know that you are hurting people around you and that you can't control yourself. It was finally necessary for me to leave work. The heat and frustration of my job were just too much for me to cope with.

My husband and I wanted very much to start a family about the time my illness began, but when I was started on Tapazole, an antithyroid drug, I was advised not to become pregnant while on this drug. This, too, made it very difficult for me to accept my disease, but I had decided on surgery as my course of treatment and felt that, hopefully, all would be cured in a few months.

I was sent to an eye doctor, who taught me how to tape my eyes shut at night. If I did not tape them, they did not quite close while I slept, which was the cause for much of their irritation. Gradually my eyes started to feel a lot better, and the emotional impact of having to tape them subsided.

I had my surgery in January, and all went well. I honestly don't remember any discomfort, except for a stiff neck. The problem that occurred was with my eyes. It was necessary for me to go to the Massachusetts Eye and Ear Infirmary for five days because of an ulcer on my cornea. This was taken care of, but I had to take cortisone pills for a month and a half to reduce the inflammation of my eyes. I was frightened over the prospect of having to stay on this medication for a long time. My vision remained blurred for a good six weeks after surgery, and this compounded my fear. The realization that I might have serious eye problems for the rest of my life was truly frightening.

It is now five years since I became ill and many things have occurred since I last wrote this account. I am still taking thyroid pills daily, but the dosage has basically been the same for years. I have my blood drawn about once a year to determine whether my dosage is too high or low. I am now so aware of what is normal that I can usually decide myself if my medication is correct or not. I no longer have to tape my eyes at night, but still use an ointment to keep them lubricated and protected in case I should open them while sleeping. I feel that I will never really look the same as I did before I developed Graves' disease, but I definitely feel that I've improved tremendously since I first got sick. When I meet new people, I no longer feel self-conscious or obligated to give an explanation about my appearance. Whenever I tell new friends about my experience, they are genuinely surprised and tell me they never noticed anything wrong with my eyes.

The most important thing to bring up-to-date about myself, however, is the fact that I have had two beautiful and healthy children since I first wrote my story. I became pregnant with my son seven months after my surgery, and he is now four years old. I also have a seven-week-old daughter, and needless to say, my husband and I are thrilled with our family. Both my pregnancies and deliveries were normal and had absolutely no complications. I had some difficulty conceiving my first child, but I honestly feel that it was because it was so soon after my thyroid surgery. I was followed very closely during both pregnancies to make sure my medication dosages were correct and my thyroid level was normal. Both children are normal and healthy and a great joy to us.

HYPERTHYROIDISM TREATED BY RADIOACTIVE IODINE

by R. D'A.

Because I had had a hysterectomy in April 1977 at age forty-nine, all my symptoms were attributed to the menopause. The subtle happenings to my system seemed natural after major surgery of this type. My pulse raced at the least exertion, and at times I had palpitations even while sitting still. I was extremely nervous, and the heat of the summer seemed more intense than in other summers. My body was always moist and clammy. Thinking this was so-called hot flashes, I tried to ignore the condition as best I could. The muscles in my arms and legs were so weak that I even had trouble opening a jar or getting out of a chair. Even climbing stairs made my legs feel tired.

As the summer moved along, other changes began to annoy me: itching eyes, shaky hands, fingernails that were wrinkled and hard to keep clean, and a steady loss of weight. I told myself it was all nerves from the sudden onset of menopause.

Finally I was hospitalized in August because of exhaustion. The nurse who admitted me said my pulse rate was 140 per minute. The doctor said she suspected a thyroid condition and ordered blood tests and a thyroid scan. The test results confirmed her suspicion: hyperthyroidism.

The doctor began to give me propylthiouracil pills to treat my condition. I was told that "PTU" (I could never remember the whole name) would slow down my thyroid and make me feel better. Sure enough, in about a week I began to feel calmer and my pulse began to slow down. By the end of a month I was almost back to normal—sweating less, no palpitations, and even a little stronger. Also, I began to gain back some of the fifteen pounds I had lost.

My doctor explained that although PTU was helping me feel better, it was likely that if I stopped the medication, my thyroid condition would probably come right back. Therefore in November I was referred to a thyroid specialist for further treatment.

For a while this new doctor had me continue the PTU, until blood tests confirmed that my thyroid level was indeed normal. He explained that because my thyroid had been overactive for a long time, and because it had not gotten smaller while I took PTU, the drug would probably not cure my condition. The doctor said that he didn't like to use

PTU for treatment for very long in someone who wasn't likey to be cured by it, because sometimes it hurt the white blood cells and might lead to an infection or other serious complications. He said that if I got an infection or fever while taking PTU, I should have a white cell count taken at my local hospital and not to start PTU again until I got a report from him. Fortunately this was never necessary.

He discussed with me the other ways my thyroid condition could be treated: surgery or "RAI" (radioactive iodine). Both treatments were fully explained. His recommendation in my particular case was RAI. I was assured of the safety of RAI, and since I had full confidence in his choice of treatment, I agreed. In December PTU was stopped for three days and a radioactive-iodine-uptake test was taken. The result was shown to me and thoroughly explained. Later that morning the doctor administered the RAI "drink," which was in a small paper cup. It was tasteless, colorless, odorless, and—best of all—painless. The most difficult part of taking the RAI was the fact that I knew it was a radioactive chemical. It was over in a few seconds, and I was on my way home.

One week later I resumed taking PTU while I waited for the radioiodine to have a chance to work completely. Ultimately I stopped the PTU and have remained completely well since then. A follow-up thyroid check once a year is all that is necessary. I do not take medication of any kind. I am now feeling great and I'm very thankful.

I have been told that my thyroid may gradually slow down sometime in the coming years, and that is the reason for my yearly "checkups." I also know that if my thyroid does slow down, I can take a thyroid pill once a day to make up the difference and keep my body healthy.

CHAPTER FIVE

The Overactive Thyroid: Other Forms of Hyperthyroidism

> I do wish to call attention to a point in support of this theory that, so far as I know, has not hitherto been made, namely, that a person 22 years of age with an adenoma of the thyroid has a definite chance of developing a train of symptoms so similar to the symptom-complex associated with hyperplastic thyroid [Graves' disease] that the best-trained diagnosticians are constantly confusing the two conditions.
>
> —From Plummer HS. The clinical and pathological relationships of Hyperplastic and Nonhyperplastic Goiter. *Journal of the American Medical Association* 1913; 61: 650.

In the preceding chapter we described a form of hyperthyroidism known as Graves' disease in which your entire thyroid gland becomes overactive. The term *hyperthyroidism* also includes several other disorders in which a greater-than-normal amount of thyroid hormone circulates in your blood stream, with the result that you may feel sick in much the same way you would if you had Graves' disease. You may get nervous and feel jumpy, dislike hot weather, and prefer cool temperatures, and you may experience attacks of rapid heart palpitations. In addition you may lose weight even though you seem to eat a normal or greater-than-normal amount of food.

The kinds of hyperthyroidism described in this chapter differ from Graves' disease in several important ways:

- Graves' disease seems to occur in individuals who have inherited a tendency or susceptibility to that condition, which is then triggered by some additional factor (such as a stressful life situation). There does not appear to be as much of an inherited tendency in these other forms of hyperthyroidism.

- For Graves' disease there is good evidence that a gradual slowing of thyroid function is part of the natural course of the disease in its late stages. Lifelong follow-up is important, to recognize and treat hypothyroidism when it occurs. Only one of these forms of hyperthyroidism (lymphocytic thyroiditis) shows this tendency to subsequent thyroid gland failure. In contrast, many of these disorders go away by themselves or can be cured completely by appropriate treatment.

- Graves' disease begins most often in women between the ages of twenty and forty. Though most of these other types of hyperthyroidism are also more common in women than men, they tend to affect people of different ages. *Toxic multinodular goiter*, for example, most commonly begins between the ages of thirty and fifty.

- Patients with Graves' disease have a tendency to develop certain other apparently related conditions. These include protrusion of the eyes (exophthalmos), lumpy skin over the shins (pretibial myxedema), and other associated autoimmune conditions (see Chapter 9). There do not seem to be similar tendencies in patients who have other forms of hyperthyroidism.

- In Graves' disease, substances known as antibodies appear in the blood and cause the thyroid to become overactive. These thyroid-stimulating antibodies do not appear to play a role in causing other forms of hyperthyroidism.

- Finally, these other kinds of hyperthyroidism are less common than Graves' disease.

With these differences in mind, we will proceed to a discussion of the important features of these other diseases that can produce hyperthyroidism.

THE HOT NODULE

Overactivity of a single thyroid nodule, actually a type of harmless thyroid tumor, accounts for about 5 percent of all hyperthyroidism. It is sometimes called a hot nodule because of its appearance in a thyroid scan (Figure 20), but it may also be referred to as *Plummer's disease* in honor of the Mayo Clinic physician who first described hyperthyroidism due to overactive nodules in 1913. Single overactive thyroid nodules are usually discovered in older women, but may occur at any age and in either sex.

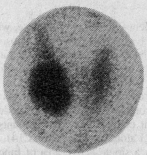

Figure 20 An overactive or "hot" nodule.

If you have diffuse toxic goiter (Graves' disease), your entire thyroid gland produces excessive amounts of thyroid hormones. If you have a hot nodule, however, only that nodule in your thyroid is functioning excessively. Gradually, as the nodule produces more and more hormone, the rest of your gland decreases its function. Finally a time is reached at which the nodule makes enough thyroid hormone to meet the needs of your whole body. But as long as the total amount of hormone made by the nodule is still "normal" for your body, you won't feel sick. It is only when the nodule makes more than enough hormone that you begin to notice symptoms of hyperthyroidism.

Sometimes a physician examining you can suspect a "hot nodule" as the cause of your hyperthyroid condition even before tests are performed. The clues to the diagnosis are the following:

- You are hyperthyroid

- Only one lump is enlarged in your thyroid, rather than the entire gland

- The rest of your thyroid gland may feel smaller than normal, since it has stopped working because your nodule is making more than enough thyroid hormone for your whole body

- Unlike a patient with Graves' disease, who often has relatives who have had a thyroid problem or other "related" conditions (see Chapter 9), if you have a hot nodule, you are less likely to have a "positive" family history

It is usually an easy matter for your doctor to prove that your hyperthyroidism is due to a hot nodule. A sample of your blood will contain increased amounts of thyroid hormone (either T3 alone or both T3 and T4), and your thyroid scan will show a single active area of function corresponding to the hot nodule (Figure 20). There will also be a drop in the amount of thyroid-stimulating hormone (TSH) released from the pituitary gland. This is a key indicator, since sometimes there is a low level of blood TSH even though your blood levels of T3 and T4 remain within the normal range. The pituitary is exquisitely sensitive to minute changes in the output of thyroid hormone from the thyroid gland and can sense that there has been an increase in hormone production even while the levels in the blood are still within the normal range. This situation, termed *subclinical hyperthyroidism*, is common in, but not unique to, patients with hot nodules; it can also be seen in patients with other forms of mild hyperthyroidism, as well as in hypothyroid patients who are taking slightly excessive quantities of thyroid hormones.

As described in Chapter 17, we are just beginning to understand why a part of your thyroid gland to become overactive in this manner, but we still don't know how to keep it from happening to you. Fortunately most patients with a hot nodule do not seem to become quite as sick as most of those who have Graves' disease. If your hot nodule does not produce hyperthyroidism, or if you have subclinical (mild) hyperthyroidism, your physician may simply examine you at periodic intervals, checking your thyroid hormone blood levels to be sure you are not developing a more severe degree of hyperthyroidism. However, your physician may feel that therapy is indicated even at a very early and mild stage.

Antithyroid drug treatment will not lead to a remission of this form of hyperthyroidism. Therefore these drugs are rarely used to treat hot nodules. If your nodule produces so much hormone that it makes you ill, your physician may advise that it be removed in an operation. Surgery should cure you, since only the nodule need be removed, and the rest of your thyroid gland can be left alone. Your normal thyroid tissue will start functioning again once the nodule has been removed, making hypothyroidism after surgery a rare occurrence.

Alternatively your physician may recommend treatment of your hot nodule with *radioactive iodine*. Radioactive iodine, usually swallowed in a capsule or drink of water, goes to your thyroid, where it is collected only by the hot nodule, since the rest of the thyroid is inactive. It remains in the nodule for several days until it is either eliminated from your body in your urine or is transformed to a nonradioactive state by a process known as *decay*. However, during its short stay in your thyroid nodule, it destroys some of the overactive thyroid tissue in the nodule. If enough tissue is destroyed or damaged in such a way that it can no longer make thyroid hormone, you will be cured. For reasons we do not understand, hot nodules usually require a larger dose of radioiodine than is needed to cure patients with Graves' disease. But in spite of the larger dose of radioactive iodine required, hypothyroidism rarely follows such treatment, since the rest of the thyroid largely escapes radiation damage. Weeks later, when your hot nodule slows its function as a result of radiation effect, the rest of your thyroid gland will start working again. You should then feel well and be permanently cured.

TOXIC MULTINODULAR GOITER

Sometimes there are several overactive nodules in your thyroid, and this is another form of Plummer's disease. This condition, known as *toxic multinodular goiter*, causes about 10 percent of all hyperthyroidism. Patients tend to be older than those who get Graves' disease, and therefore they may get sicker from the rapid pulse, weakness, and weight loss that occur because of the high level of thyroid hormone. In most cases a goiter has been present for many years, gradually becoming more and more overactive until hyperthyroidism develops.

If you have a toxic multinodular goiter, your physician may suspect this condition because you will have symptoms of hyperthyroidism and an enlarged, lumpy-feeling thyroid gland. The diagnosis is usually confirmed by a blood test that shows a high level of thyroid hormone and a low level of TSH, and by a thyroid scan that demonstrates several areas of increased thyroid activity (Figure 21).

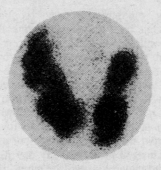

Figure 21 Multinodular goiter.

We don't know what causes multinodular goiters to become hyperactive. In rare cases a person with a nodular goiter abruptly develops hyperthyroidism after taking an iodine-containing drug such as *amiodarone*, used to treat heart-rhythm disturbances, or after an X ray that uses iodine-containing contrast material to enhance the images, such as a CAT scan or kidney X ray. More commonly, however, if hyperthyroidism develops, it is a gradual process that occurs over many years. Therefore your physician will need to check your thyroid function only once or twice a year. Like the situation with hot nodules, treatment of this form of hyperthyroidism is usually straightforward. If you are sick because of the high level of thyroid hormone in your system when you first see your physician, your symptoms can be helped promptly with a *beta-adrenergic blocking drug*, such as atenolol or propanolol, which blocks the action of the hormone on your body, slowing your pulse and generally making you feel better. In addition an antithyroid drug such as propylthiouracil or methimazole (Tapazole) can be used to slow down production of hormone by the overactive thyroid nodules. But since toxic multinodular goiter does not tend to subside by itself (as sometimes occurs in Graves' disease), permanent control of the condition is unlikely unless your physician decreases the number of overactive cells in your thyroid gland.

This may be accomplished by radioactive iodine treatment, but the effects of treatment are slightly different from those encountered with a hot nodule. Since the radioiodine goes into several overactive parts of your thyroid, it is more possible that you will become hypothyroid sometime in the future. Similarly if thyroid surgery is chosen for your toxic multinodular goiter, the surgeon will probably remove most of the thyroid gland, making hypothyroidism after surgery more likely. If too much tissue is left behind, your hyperthyroidism may recur, since new nodules may develop and produce excessive amounts of the hormone.

By either method the hyperthyroidism can be safely controlled, and if hypothyroidism results from the treatment, it is a simple matter to raise your thyroid-hormone blood level to normal with thyroid hormone tablets taken once a day. Your physician will probably want to test your thyroid periodically in the years that follow, since overactive nodules may reappear and change the level of thyroid hormone in your system, possibly even causing hyperthyroidism again. If that happens, the principles of treatment will be the same as before, and usually will involve the use of radioactive iodine.

HYPERTHYROIDISM ASSOCIATED WITH THYROID INFLAMMATION

Sometimes, in association with a viral infection, a form of thyroid inflammation known as *subacute thyroiditis* develops. If you have subacute thyroiditis, you may think you have the flu or a very bad sore throat, for you will probably have fever, ache all over, and have a very sore neck because of your tender, inflamed thyroid gland (Figure 22).

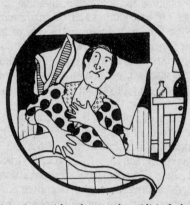

Figure 22 A patient with subacute thyroiditis feels sick and has a tender, inflamed thyroid.

Thyroid hormone tends to leak out of the inflamed gland, and if enough gets into your system, symptoms of hyperthyroidism may appear. Since your thyroid is not overactive, your doctor can identify this form of hyperthyroidism because you will have an elevated blood level of thyroid hormone and a low TSH level, yet a low radioiodine uptake by the thyroid gland (proof of the gland's inactivity). A high *red blood cell sedimentation rate* is another essential factor helping your doctor make this diagnosis, for it reflects the degree of thyroid inflammation. Since the disease is self-limited, treatment with aspirin or similar drugs for your sore neck, fever, and aching muscles and a beta-adrenergic blocking drug like atenolol or propanolol for your symptoms of hyperthyroidism are usually sufficient. Prompt improvement can be expected, and complete cure should follow within two to three months. Sometimes treatment with cortisone is needed because of inadequate control of the symptoms by aspirin. A period of hypothyroidism can follow the hyperthyroid phase of this illness. This usually is mild, lasts no more than a month, and represents the time it takes for your thyroid to start working again. If you feel sluggish and tired because of the low thyroid-hormone level, your physician may prescribe thyroid-hormone tablets, but usually this is not necessary.

Lymphocytic thyroiditis is a condition that has only recently been recognized. When the disease occurs after pregnancy, it is called *postpartum thyroiditis*. In various reports from around the United States, this occurs in about 8 percent of women after childbirth. It shares many of the features of hyperthyroidism associated with subacute thyroiditis: Patients have high blood levels of thyroid hormones but a low radioiodine uptake. Unlike most patients with subacute thyroiditis, however, patients with this condition do not have a painful thyroid gland or a very high red blood cell sedimentation rate. In short they lack the symptoms and signs of thyroid inflammation.

If you develop this condition you will be treated as if you had subacute thyroiditis, except that you won't need aspirin since the disease is not painful. Usually your physician will control your hyperthyroid symptoms with a drug such as atenolol or propranolol until the disease subsides spontaneously in a few weeks. A transient period of hypothyroidism usually follows the hyperthyroidism, similar to that seen in subacute thyroiditis. Treatment is rarely required in this circumstance. Recent studies suggest that this form of hyperthyroidism may be followed by temporary or occasionally permanent thyroid failure either immediately after the hyperthyroidism or some time later in life, so periodic checkups are important if you have had spontaneously resolving hyperthyroidism. (See Chapter 7 for more information.)

HYPERTHYROIDISM CAUSED BY IODINE

It has been known for many years that iodine can cause hyperthyroidism in certain susceptible individuals, but the reasons for this curious phenomenon are unknown. Before 1972 the problem was seen only in iodine-deficient areas of the world. When needed dietary iodine supplements were introduced into the food in those areas, some of the inhabitants developed hyperthyroidism. Sometimes the hyperthyroidism went away by itself, but usually it had to be controlled by drugs, radioactive iodine, or thyroid surgery.

More recently we have learned that excessive iodine may cause hyperthyroidism even in individuals who have normal amounts of iodine in their diets. Excessive iodine might come from iodine in foods such as kelp (seaweed), in medications such as expectorants or the heart medicine amiodarone, or in X-ray dyes such as those used in a CAT scan or to X-ray the kidneys, gall bladder, spinal canal, or blood vessels. Patients with underlying nodular goiters are the ones most likely to experience this "thyrotoxic" effect of iodine.

If you have hyperthyroidism due to excessive iodine, your physician will first try to see that your extra iodine intake is stopped. Second, your symptoms will probably be controlled with atenolol, propranolol, or one of the other beta-adrenergic blocking drugs until it is determined whether your thyroid overactivity will subside spontaneously. If you remain hyperthyroid, other measures can be taken. Your treatment may include antithyroid drugs as well as surgical removal of the thyroid gland. Radioactive iodine treatment is not successful for this condition because the excess iodine already present in your system dilutes the therapeutic effect of the radioactive iodine.

OVERMEDICATION WITH THYROID HORMONE

Hyperthyroidism may occur in anyone who is taking too much thyroid hormone. Emotionally disturbed patients have been known to take too much hormone intentionally; they are best advised to seek help for their problem rather than hurt themselves with medicine. On the other hand this kind of problem is sometimes observed in individuals who have no intention of causing themselves trouble. It may seem obvious that you should not take too much thyroid hormone or the wrong kind of thyroid hormone, but we are now learning that it is not always so simple. Medical studies show that if your own thyroid gland is underactive, you probably require a daily dose of no more than 100 to 200 micrograms of thyroxine as adequate replacement therapy.

If you are taking more than this amount of thyroxine, you may have symptoms of hyperthyroidism due to the medication itself. Your physician can tell whether your thyroid-hormone dosage is correct or excessive by measuring the amount of TSH in your blood. If you are overmedicated, your blood TSH level will be low. In that case your dosage can be gradually reduced until your blood level of TSH normalizes, indicating that your pituitary gland senses that there is now the correct amount of thyroid hormone in your system. Once your thyroid-hormone requirements are known, your physician may not check your thyroid-hormone and TSH levels more than once a year.

TUMORS THAT CAN CAUSE HYPERTHYROIDISM

Several kinds of tumors have been found to be an occasional cause of hyperthyroidism. Thyroid cancer is one such tumor. Sometimes thyroid-cancer cells are able to make thyroid hormone, and when there are enough cells present in your body, hyperthyroidism may occur.

Very rarely tumors in other parts of the body can influence your thyroid. For example, there are several hundred reports of patients in whom pituitary gland tumors have made excessive amounts of TSH. Here treatment is usually best directed against the pituitary (which is the real culprit), rather than against the thyroid, which, in this instance, is an innocent bystander. Other rare tumors that have caused hyperthyroidism have occurred in the reproductive system. When they are recognized, they are dealt with directly through treatment aimed at the source of the problem.

CHAPTER SIX

The Underactive Thyroid:
Hypothyroidism and Myxedema

Mrs. S., aged 46, was shown at a meeting of the Northumberland and Durham Medical Society on February 12th, 1891.... At the time of this meeting she presented the typical features of an advanced case of myxedema.... The experimental nature of the treatment was explained, and the patient, realizing the otherwise hopeless outlook, promptly consented to this trial.... The thyroid gland was removed from a freshly killed sheep with sterilized instruments and conveyed at once in a sterilized bottle to the laboratory where the glycerine extract was prepared.... In the treatment of this case, a hypodermic injection of 25 minims of extract was given twice a week at first, and later on at longer intervals. The patient steadily improved, and three months later ... the condition was thus described:

"The swelling has gradually diminished ... and the face ... has greatly improved in appearance and has much more expression, as many of the natural wrinkles have returned. The speech has become more rapid and fluent ... she answers questions much more readily, the mind has become more active, and the memory has improved. She is more active in all her movements and finds that it requires much less effort than formerly to do her housework ... the skin has been much less dry and she perspires when walking ... she is no longer sensitive to cold.... After this, the injections were given at fortnightly intervals, and later on ... she took 10 minims by mouth six nights a week. The patient was then enabled to live in good health for over twenty-eight years after she had reached an advanced stage of myxedema. During this period she consumed over nine pints of liquid thyroid extract or its equivalent, prepared from the thyroid glands of more than 870 sheep."

—From Murray GR. Life-history of the first case of Myxedema Treated by Thyroid Extract. *British Medical Journal* 1920; 1:359.
The patient was treated from 1891 until her death in 1919.

When the thyroid gland fails to produce a normal amount of thyroid hormone, a condition known as hypothyroidism results. In a survey done many years ago at several large hospitals, less than one patient in a thousand was reported as having hypothyroidism, so it was assumed to be a relatively uncommon disorder. Recently an improved method for identifying mild degrees of thyroid failure using the serum TSH has revealed that the true incidence of hypothyroidism in the population is much higher. For example a recent survey found elevated blood levels of thyroid-stimulating hormone (TSH) in seventy-five of every thousand women (7.5 percent) and twenty-eight of every thousand men (2.8 percent) tested. Other large-population surveys have shown that primary thyroid-gland failure is more common in women than in men by almost fourfold. In addition the condition affects older people more commonly than it does younger individuals. For example, 15 to 20 percent of women and 5 to 10 percent of men over the age of sixty years will have mild or severe thyroid gland failure. Most physicians believe that elevated TSH levels represent the earliest sign of thyroid failure, since many patients with an elevated TSH will go on to develop more evidence of hypothyroidism. Specifically, 20 to 100 percent of individuals with mild thyroid-gland failure will advance to more severe hypothyroidism within four years, depending on age, sex, and other factors.

Thyroid hormones act upon receptors in tissues throughout your body. Therefore it is not surprising that the complaints that you develop in hypothyroidism may involve many different parts of your system. Thyroid hormones control the rate at which various things happen, such as the speed of chemical reactions, the rate of tissue growth, and the rate at which electrical impulses travel in your nerves and muscles. So when you become hypothyroid, many of the affected bodily functions simply slow down.

As your thyroid begins to fail, you may feel perfectly well, for often the only suggestion of a problem will be a slight enlargement of your thyroid gland (goiter), appearing as a lump or swelling in front of your neck. Then, as your thyroid-hormone level falls farther, you may begin to feel tired and listless, perhaps chilly when those about you are comfortably warm. As your skin, hair, and fingernails grow more slowly, they become thickened, dry, and brittle. Some hair loss may be noticed. Then, as your hypothyroidism becomes more severe, changes may occur in the tissues beneath your skin that lead to a characteristic puffy, swollen appearance known as myxedema. This is often particularly apparent around your face and eyes.

Your circulation is affected and your heart rate slows, but you probably won't notice this unless someone happens to count your pulse (it may be below 60 beats per minute). Since your intestinal activity slows down, you may become constipated. A few pounds of weight gain may occur due to water retention, but you are not likely to get fat due to hypothyroidism alone because your appetite and zest for food decreases when you become hypothyroid. Your muscles may become sore and you may be awakened at night with leg cramps. Muscle swelling may occur and may make your tongue (which is a muscle) bigger. Your nervous system may be affected in several ways. You may notice some memory loss, decreased ability to think, or depression, and you may become more sensitive to medications, so that weak sedatives cause prolonged sleep. Some patients experience tingling in their fingers, or loss of balance and difficulty in walking.

If you are a younger woman, changes in your reproductive system may cause longer, heavier, and more frequent menstruation. Your ovaries may stop producing an egg each month and, if so, it may be difficult for you to get pregnant. If pregnancy does occur, you are a little more likely to have a miscarriage than if you had a healthy thyroid.

In summary, if you become hypothyroid, the most common complaint you are likely to have is feeling "rundown." You will feel as though you are running on one or two cylinders rather than six or eight. However, subtle changes are probably occurring all over your body as a result of your low thyroid-hormone levels.

WHAT CAUSES HYPOTHYROIDISM?

The causes of hypothyroidism vary somewhat with the age at which the disorder begins. Most children born with severe hypothyroidism have never developed enough thyroid tissue to supply adequate amounts of thyroid hormones for their bodily needs. Other hypothyroid infants may have an inherited defect in the production of thyroid hormones within their thyroid gland. In some underdeveloped countries dietary iodine deficiency is an important added cause of serious hypothyroidism and cretinism in newborn babies. Although iodine deficiency is no longer a problem in the United States, the opposite condition—iodine excess in pregnancy—still does occur. If a woman consumes too much iodine (usually in medication) during pregnancy, the result may be that her unborn baby's thyroid slows its production of thyroid hormone in the presence of the extra iodine. If so, her baby may be born with hypothyroidism and a goiter.

In older children and adults a silent, ongoing inflammation (without evidence of infection) of the thyroid, known as chronic lymphocytic thyroiditis (also known as Hashimoto's disease, in honor of the Japanese physician who described it), is the most common cause of thyroid gland failure. The thyroid fails because inflammation and scarring damage the thyroid tissue. At some point enough tissue will have been destroyed so that whatever remains can no longer produce an adequate amount of thyroid hormone to meet the body's needs. (See Chapter 7 for a more complete discussion of thyroiditis.) This disorder is most likely due to an autoimmune process in which the body's immune system attacks the thyroid gland and destroys it. This type of hypothyroidism most frequently appears after age fifty.

Thyroid failure is also very common among patients who have been treated in the past for an overactive thyroid. Here, hypothyroidism may occur immediately after a treatment that destroys or removes part of the thyroid (radioactive iodine or an operation), but in most instances the thyroid doesn't fail until months or years later. Such a delayed onset of hypothyroidism suggests that the original treatment is not the only cause of thyroid failure in such patients. Coexistent chronic lymphocytic thyroiditis may be a factor as well.

Less commonly the thyroid may fail temporarily after a viral infection (see the discussion of subacute thyroiditis, Chapter 7) or because of a medication. For example if an antithyroid drug used to control an overactive thyroid is given in too large a dose, hypothyroidism may result and last until the dosage of that drug is reduced. Lithium, a psychiatric drug, can also cause hypothyroidism in some people. Furthermore some individuals have thyroid glands that are very sensitive to iodine. They can develop hypothyroidism as a side effect if they are given iodine in a medication such as amiodarone. Health food users can similarly, and unknowingly, take in excessive amounts of iodine by eating seaweed *(dulse)* or kelp. Hypothyroidism can also develop in patients who receive large amounts of X rays to the neck area as part of cancer treatment.

DIAGNOSING HYPOTHYROIDISM

If your physician suspects hypothyroidism, he or she will first perform a medical examination to look for evidence that your thyroid level is low. The most important test in making a certain diagnosis of this condition is your TSH blood level. When your thyroid gland fails, your pituitary begins to produce increased amounts of TSH in an effort to stimulate your thyroid and return it to normal function. If your thyroid is damaged, it cannot increase its activity, and your blood level of TSH rises and remains high. Detecting an increased level of TSH in your blood also provides helpful evidence that your hypothyroidism is due to disease within your thyroid gland and is not a result of inadequate stimulation of your thyroid by a diseased pituitary gland.

A word should be said about a dangerous recent trend in the lay press to minimize the importance of thyroid blood tests in the diagnosis and management of hypothyroidism. The thyroid tests available twenty or thirty years ago were simply not specific and sensitive enough to tell if a person was truly hypothyroid. Today, however, very accurate and relatively inexpensive tests are available, and they should always be used by your physician to help make a diagnosis of hypothyroidism. Such a diagnosis should never be based solely on complaints of weight gain, fatigue, or infertility, or on such nonspecific findings as dry skin or a low body temperature. Well-informed physicians do not start patients on thyroid medication until blood tests, most importantly the TSH blood level test, confirming the diagnosis are obtained. Blood tests are essential in determining the cause and severity of the hypothyroidism, and in assessing the adequacy of thyroid therapy. The level of the thyroid hormones (T4 and T3) may also be checked, but these tests are less useful than the TSH level in making the diagnosis of primary hypothyroidism, though they may be helpful in estimating the dose of medication that you might require.

Finally, since most hypothyroidism is caused by chronic lymphocytic thyroiditis, a sample of your blood can be checked for the antibodies that may appear as a clue to the presence of this type of thyroid inflammation.

THE TREATMENT OF HYPOTHYROIDISM

Hypothyroidism is treated with thyroid-hormone tablets containing precisely the same chemical compound that your thyroid normally produces and therefore you will not be allergic to it. Moreover the hormones are not destroyed by stomach juices, so they can be taken orally. Finally, if administered correctly, thyroid hormone has no unwanted effects on any body tissues.

Today many different thyroid-hormone preparations are manufactured. For many years, however, the only thyroid-hormone medications available were made from animal thyroid glands. These preparations were very useful, but unfortunately they contain not only thyroxine (T4) but also a second more rapidly acting thyroid hormone, triiodothyronine (T3). We prefer to administer thyroid-hormone tablets that do not contain T3 for two reasons. First, the body normally makes T3 from T4; in fact much of our T4 is changed into T3 under normal circumstances as it is used by the body. Second, the blood T3 level can become abnormally high after taking medication that contains T3. The abnormally high T3 level can cause a rapid pulse and increase the workload of the heart, which can be dangerous for anyone with underlying heart disease. For these reasons most physicians now treat hypothyroidism with tablets of pure T4.

There is an increasing tendency today to use generic forms of drugs as opposed to more expensive forms sold under a trade name. Although generic drugs are generally less expensive, generic thyroid preparations have always presented a problem of unreliable potency. Recently tests conducted in the United States have shown this variability of potency in generic T4 tablets. In fact only three kinds of T4 tablets are found to be consistently reliable: Synthroid, Levothroid, and Levoxyl. Therefore the authors prescribe only these thyroid preparations at this time. These tablets have a nearly identical "color code" (thyroxine tablets of different potencies come in different colors), which helps to avoid confusion about thyroid-hormone dosage. A wide variety of dosage strengths are available to enable the physician to precisely tailor the dose to the patient (table 1).

TABLE 1

Comparative Availability of Thyroxine Preparations in the United States and Canada

Tablet Color Available as

Thyroxine Dosage (in micrograms)	Synthroid	Levoxyl	Levothroid	Eltroxin
25	orange	orange	orange	———
50	white	white	white	white
75	violet	purple	gray	———
88	olive	olive	mint green	———
100	yellow	yellow	yellow	yellow
112	rose	rose	rose	———
125	brown	brown	purple	———
137	———	dark blue	blue	———
150	blue	blue	light blue	blue
175	lilac	turquoise	turquoise	———
200	pink	pink	pink	pink
300	green	green	lime green	green

Synthroid is available in the United States and Canada. Levoxyl and Levothroid are available only in the United States, and Eltroxin only in Canada.

When thyroxine tablets first began to be used, physicians thought that 100 micrograms of T4 was equivalent in potency to a one-grain tablet of desiccated thyroid, or Proloid. In practice, however, we have found that these older preparations are not reliably potent. Therefore when changing a patient from a desiccated thyroid tablet to T4, we usually start at a slightly lower dose of T4. For example someone who has taken two or three grains of thyroid may be started on 75 to 125 micrograms of thyroxine. In fact few patients ever need more than 100 to 200 micrograms of thyroxine per day.

Certain drugs can interfere with the absorption of thyroxin from your intestine. These include cholestyramine (Questran) and cholestipol (Colestid) used to treat high cholesterol, aluminum hydroxide (an antacid), sucralfate (Carafate) used to treat stomach ulcers, and probably iron supplements used to treat anemia. If you take any of these medications, it is important that you take your thyroid tablet several hours before or after these other medications to ensure that all the thyroid hormone is absorbed into your system.

Even when hypothyroidism is severe, a few months of thyroid treatment should lead to complete recovery and a return to good health. At that time your physician will probably measure your blood levels of T4 and TSH to be sure that your dosage of thyroid hormone is correct. If you are taking too much T4, your blood level of TSH will be too low and the blood level of T4 may be above the normal range. On the other hand, if your dose of T4 is too low, your blood level of TSH will still be high and the T4 level may be low.

Don't Stop Taking Your Thyroid Medication

The smooth control of thyroid-hormone levels that physicians achieve by using pure thyroxine preparations is due to the slow rate at which thyroxine is used up by the body. In fact if a normal person's thyroid suddenly stopped working, it would take about seven days for the body to use up just half of the T4 already in the blood. Therefore if you are hypothyroid and taking thyroxine tablets to correct your thyroid deficiency, you will not feel suddenly sick even if you stop your thyroxine tablets abruptly. Furthermore because you won't notice a sudden change in the way you feel, you may incorrectly assume that your thyroid condition no longer exists, and you may stop taking your medication entirely. Unfortunately when your hypothyroidism does recur, its onset may be so gradual that you may not realize that you are becoming ill again until your symptoms are pronounced.

In hypothyroidism due to chronic lymphocytic thyroiditis, there is also a need for good "family follow-up" since this illness, like hyperthyroidism due to Graves' disease, is a genetically transmitted disease. The genes for it came from either your mother or your father (rarely from both). Therefore older members on the side of the family affected should be checked for thyroid problems as well as for certain associated medical conditions. These relationships are discussed in Chapter 8.

If you are hypothyroid, it is important that you see your physician periodically for checkups. Since most hypothyroidism tends to get progressively worse over time, a dose of thyroid hormone that was correct several years ago may well be inadequate as thyroid replacement now. Therefore your physician will probably want to measure your serum T4 and TSH periodically to be sure that a change in hormone dosage is not indicated. We recommend that patients should be tested at least once each year to be sure that the control of the thyroid condition is correct. An exception to this rule applies if you become pregnant. Pregnancy often increases the thyroid-hormone requirement. Therefore if you become pregnant while taking thyroid hormone for hypothyroidism, we recommend that you have your TSH level checked two months into the pregnancy. If the value is high, your doctor will increase your dose of medication until you have safely delivered your child. Then your dose will be reduced to the previous level.

A word might be said about treating certain of the less common causes of thyroid failure. For example, subacute thyroiditis, which may be due to a viral infection, may only temporarily decrease thyroid function. If a patient needs any thyroxine treatment for a transient hypothyroid condition, it should be only a matter of weeks or months before he or she can stop the drug and remain well. And when hypothyroidism is due to iodine ingestion or an antithyroid drug, simply stopping or decreasing the dose of the drug may be all that is required. In every such instance your physician has the necessary tests available as a guide in properly taking care of you. A very special example of this is the hypothyroidism that occurs soon after delivering a child. This condition, known as postpartum thyroiditis, is found in approximately 5 to 8 percent of all women in the postpartum period. It usually develops two to six months after delivery and commonly requires treatment with thyroid hormone. Surprisingly this form of hypothyroidism is usually not permanent and goes away spontaneously after six to twelve months. Thus for this type of hypothyroidism your doctor will discontinue the thyroid medication after a few months to see if the problem has disappeared. However, hypothyroidism is permanent in about 25 percent of women with this disorder.

As we have already suggested, many patients who were started on thyroid medication years ago may not have needed thyroid treatment then, and may not need it now. Thyroid testing available today makes it possible for us to find out safely and easily whether such patients can stop their thyroid tablets and remain well.

If you took thyroid-hormone treatment for many years and want to know if you still need the medication, please ask your physician for guidance rather than stopping treatment on your own. If you both agree to a trial without thyroid tablets, your physician will probably measure your blood level of TSH four to six weeks after you have stopped the medication. If your TSH level is normal, you do not need further thyroxine treatment, for your own thyroid function is fine. If that is your situation, your physician will probably recheck your thyroid function with a TSH test after several months to be sure your thyroid remains healthy.

OTHER KINDS OF HYPOTHYROIDISM

Since the pituitary gland at the base of your brain controls and stimulates your thyroid, a tumor or other problem that involves the pituitary can cause secondary thyroid failure. Since your pituitary also controls other glands, including

your reproductive organs and adrenal glands, it is usually
an easy matter for your physician to tell if this is the case.
For example, a woman with secondary (pituitary) hypothyroidism will usually stop menstruating when her diseased
pituitary gland stops stimulating her ovaries properly. Physicians have at their disposal both X-ray techniques and
laboratory tests to evaluate the function of your pituitary
gland as well as your thyroid. If there is indeed a pituitary
problem, you will probably require treatment for other hormonal deficiencies in addition to the thyroid. If your pituitary fails because of a tumor, specific treatment may be
directed at the pituitary gland itself. Fortunately pituitary tumors respond to both surgical and radiation treatment. Just
as with primary hypothyroidism, you will need careful and
prolonged follow-up, for in addition to thyroid-hormone requirements, the amounts of other hormones you take may
vary with time. Thus periodic blood tests and X rays of the
pituitary area will probably be recommended by your physician.

The pituitary is itself under the control of the *hypothalamus*, an even higher center within the brain. In very rare
instances disease in the region of the hypothalamus has
caused the pituitary to fail and in turn has caused thyroid
and other glandular problems. Although this condition
looks very much like secondary hypothyroidism, physicians
can usually distinguish one form from another by means of
careful testing. Treatment is similar to that given when the
problem is in the pituitary gland, and it must include correction not only of the hypothyroidism but also of the other
glandular deficiencies as well.

A rare form of hypothyroidism has been found in a few
families in which the body tissues do not have a normal
ability to respond to thyroid hormone. This inherited condition is called *generalized resistance to thyroid hormone*. In
this situation the thyroid gland produces plenty of thyroid
hormone. In fact blood levels are increased above normal,
yet the body cannot respond because of an abnormality in
tissue thyroid-hormone receptors. Since the pituitary gland
is one of the tissues that does not respond normally to thyroid hormone, the blood level of TSH in these individuals
is increased, despite high T4 levels. Even though patients

who have this condition usually look and act normally, we now know that children with this problem are likely to be hyperactive, and up to 70 percent of them may experience attention deficit disorders. As of 1995 over one hundred families have been found to have this problem. Fortunately the unusual combination of high thyroid-hormone levels and high/normal TSH levels should make this problem easy for physicians to recognize.

SUMMARY

Hypothyroidism is almost always due to disease within your thyroid gland that causes a decrease in the production of thyroid hormone. The most common cause of this disorder is autoimmune thyroid disease, which is transmitted genetically and affects women much more often than men. Excellent tests, particularly the blood TSH level, are available to diagnose the condition accurately, and treatment with thyroxine should restore you to good health. Because the condition runs in families, some of your relatives should be checked for thyroid problems by their own physicians (see Chapter 8).

CHAPTER SEVEN

Inflammation of the Thyroid:
Hashimoto's Disease and Other Forms of Thyroiditis

Thyroiditis is the general term used to describe several different disorders in which the thyroid gland becomes inflamed. Most commonly the inflammation takes the form of a chronic, progressive disease known as chronic lymphocytic thyroiditis or *Hashimoto's disease* (in honor of the Japanese physician who, in 1912, first described the microscopic changes in the thyroid tissue of patients with the condition). Patients with this form of thyroiditis sometimes exhibit so few symptoms that the disease may go unnoticed for many years, but eventually it may destroy so much thyroid tissue that hypothyroidism develops.

Lymphocytic thyroiditis may also occur as a self-limited condition that lasts two to six months, resolving spontaneously and leaving most patients with normal thyroid function. When it occurs after pregnancy, it is termed *postpartum thyroiditis*. Another painless variant of lymphocytic thyroiditis may occur at other times and has been termed *silent thyroiditis*.

Subacute thyroiditis or *deQuervain's disease*, is another condition caused by thyroid inflammation, one that is distinct from those mentioned above. The disease often seems to follow the course of a viral infection. The thyroid gland is usually painful and looks quite different on microscopic examination.

Finally, *very* rarely the thyroid may become suddenly and dramatically inflamed with a bacterial infection. This condition is referred to as *acute suppurative thyroiditis*.

Since these various forms of thyroiditis are completely separate disorders—each with different causes, clinical courses, and treatments—they will be considered individually.

CHRONIC LYMPHOCYTIC THYROIDITIS
(HASHIMOTO'S DISEASE)

Hashimoto's disease appears to be an inherited condition. As with Graves' disease, you probably must inherit a gene or set of genes to be *able* to develop this disorder. However, even though you may inherit this genetic tendency, you still may never actually develop the disease itself. Therefore there must be other factors that cause this condition to develop.

These other factors include gender, age, and your body's immune system. Thus women are affected about four to eight times more often than men. Although you may develop this form of thyroiditis in childhood or adolescence, it is most commonly diagnosed after the age of fifty, for this is when affected patients usually become hypothyroid. As described in Chapter 3, your body's immune system plays a role in the production of the thyroid inflammation and tissue destruction that occurs in chronic lymphocytic thyroiditis. Substances known as *autoantibodies*, made by white blood cells called *lymphocytes*, appear in your blood in this condition. Although we do not yet fully understand how or why these lymphocytes and antibodies work, the final result is damage to thyroid tissue. When enough tissue has been destroyed, your thyroid-hormone production falls below normal, and symptoms of hypothyroidism appear.

This form of thyroiditis is common, and its incidence may well be increasing. A population survey in Minnesota carried out by physicians at the Mayo Clinic between 1935 and 1944 reported that, among women, new cases of chronic lymphocytic thyroiditis occurred at a rate of 6.5 per 100,000 women per year. When the same Minnesota population group was studied again in 1965–67, this "annual incidence" of the disorder had increased to 69 per 100,000 women per year.

One way that physicians have tried to estimate the prevalence of Hashimoto's disease is by testing large populations of people for hypothyroidism. As noted above, this form of thyroiditis damages thyroid tissue and leads to thyroid failure. The most sensitive test for hypothyroidism is a blood test that measures the level of the pituitary's thyroid-stimulating hormone (TSH). When TSH tests are carried out on large numbers of people, we find that about 10 percent of women and 4 percent of men over the age of fifty have an elevated blood level of TSH. By age sixty TSH is increased in as many as 15 to 20 percent of women and 5 to 10 percent of men. Put another way, at least one woman in six and one man in twelve will develop Hashimoto's disease in his or her lifetime. Each could potentially develop subsequent hypothyroidism and should be watched for signs of thyroid failure.

If you develop this condition, your thyroid inflammation will probably be so mild that at first you won't even know that anything is wrong. The first indication of a problem may be a goiter: You may develop a gradual painless enlargement of your thyroid gland. During this period your thyroid gland is becoming infiltrated with lymphocytes, which start gradual thyroid destruction and scarring that may result in subsequent thyroid failure. If the function of your thyroid decreases to the point that your gland can no longer make a normal amount of thyroid hormone, symptoms of hypothyroidism appear, and you may begin to look and feel sick for the first time. At this point the destruction of your thyroid may be so extensive that very little normal thyroid tissue remains.

When hypothyroidism occurs, you will probably feel sluggish and "run-down," but the disease progresses slowly, so you may not realize that anything is wrong. Constipation, leg cramps, hair loss, and mental dullness may appear, together with other symptoms and signs of thyroid failure already outlined in Chapter 6. However, since chronic lymphocytic thyroiditis tends to be a progressive condition, your thyroid-hormone level will probably continue to fall, causing your symptoms of hypothyroidism to worsen until your disease is recognized and treated.

If you visit your doctor and appear to have hypothyroidism, a goiter, and no history of a past problem with your thyroid, your physician will probably suspect that you have chronic lymphocytic thyroiditis. This diagnosis becomes even more likely if other members of your family have had overactive or underactive thyroids. Your physician can confirm the presence of hypothyroidism by means of a blood test that shows a low level of thyroid hormone (T4) and a high blood level of thyroid-stimulating hormone (TSH). The elevated TSH level is the more important test, for it is more sensitive and proves that your thyroid, not your pituitary, has failed (see Chapter 6). Also, a blood test demonstrating the presence of antithyroid antibodies provides strong evidence of thyroiditis.

Since thyroiditis occurs throughout the gland, a radioiodine scan of your thyroid merely confirms the generalized nature of the process by showing a patchy uptake of radioiodine throughout the gland (Figure 23). Such a scan is not usually needed to diagnose or to plan treatment for this condition, so your physician is not likely to order this test, thus saving you an unnecessary expense. On the other hand your physician may recommend a scan if your thyroid contains one or more lumps (nodules), which can occur in lymphocytic thyroiditis. Cancerous nodules do not concentrate radioiodine (Figure 24), so if your thyroid contains a nodule that appears "cold," or nonfunctional, on scan, more tests, including a biopsy of the nodule, should be performed to be sure that cancer is not present.

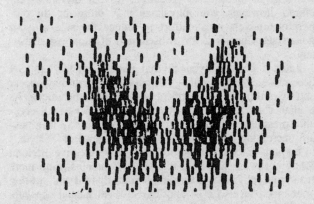

Figure 23   A thyroid scan of a patient with chronic lymphocytic thyroiditis usually shows a patchy pattern of radioiodine throughout the thyroid.

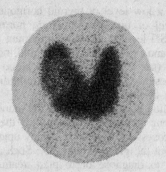

Figure 24 An inactive or "cold" nodule.

Absolute proof of the presence of chronic lymphocytic thyroiditis can be obtained through a biopsy of your thyroid gland and microscopic examination of the tissue. Fortunately a biopsy is rarely necessary, since the other tests we have discussed usually provide your physician with enough information to make the diagnosis.

In the early stages of this condition, while your thyroid hormone levels and TSH remain normal, you should feel well and no treatment is required. If your thyroid is enlarged, however, your physician may prescribe thyroid-hormone tablets in an effort to reduce the size of your goiter (see Chapter 2 for a discussion of suppression therapy).

Later, if and when your thyroid gland fails and your TSH becomes elevated symptoms of hypothyroidism may appear and thyroid hormone treatment is likely to be beneficial. As explained in detail in Chapter 6, your physician will probably prescribe thyroxine (T4) tablets once a day in gradually increasing dosages until your blood level of TSH falls to normal. Since this condition may be progressive, lifelong follow-up is essential, but this usually amounts to no more than your physician examining your thyroid and testing your blood levels of T4 and TSH at your annual checkup. As your thyroid gland's function declines, your thyroid-hormone dosage may be increased appropriately. On the other hand the dosage may actually decrease in some elderly persons because the body's need for thyroid hormone often decreases as people grow older.

OTHER FORMS OF LYMPHOCYTIC THYROIDITIS

Several other types of thyroiditis seem to cause the same type of thyroid inflammation, judging by the microscopic appearance of the involved thyroid tissue. They are presented separately from Hashimoto's disease because these diseases have other characteristics that distinguish them from the more common, chronic form of lymphocytic thyroiditis.

Postpartum Thyroiditis

A woman's immune system is suppressed during pregnancy, but becomes more active following delivery of a baby (see Chapter 13 for a more detailed explanation). If you have a genetic tendency toward autoimmune thyroid problems, you may experience a painless inflammation of the thyroid as your immune system becomes more active in the months after delivery, even if you have no history of thyroid problems before or during pregnancy. In its early stages hyperthyroid symptoms may occur if excessive amounts of thyroid hormone leak into the blood stream from your inflamed thyroid gland. Later on, when the thyroid's supply of hormones is exhausted, blood levels of these hormones often fall below normal, and symptoms of hypothyroidism may appear (Figure 25).

Beta-adrenergic blocking drugs such as propranolol, atenolol, and metoprolol are usually enough to control the symptoms if you develop hyperthyroidism in the early weeks of this condition. If your thyroid fails after several months, supplementary thyroid-hormone tablets can be given to maintain blood levels in the normal range.

Although complete recovery is common, about 25 percent of all women with postpartum thyroiditis progress to permanent hypothyroidism within three to four years, and require lifelong treatment.

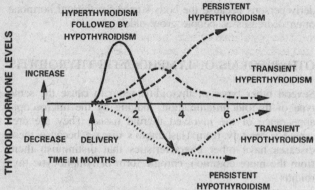

Figure 25   Thyroid dysfunction after pregnancy.

Often there is so much going on in a new mother's life that postpartum thyroiditis goes unrecognized or is mistaken for postpartum depression. Some physicians feel that all pregnant women should be given a screening antithyroid antibody blood test in early pregnancy to identify those who are at risk for this condition; if it is positive, a TSH blood test to evaluate thyroid function should be performed in the postpartum period. See Chapter 13 for more discussion of this and other important points about this condition.

Silent Thyroiditis (Spontaneously Resolving Hyperthyroidism)

Transient lymphocytic thyroiditis may also develop at times other than the postpartum period. Beginning in the early 1970s physicians in the midwestern United States noted an increasing incidence of cases of hyperthyroidism that, like postpartum thyroiditis, was associated with a low radioactive-iodine uptake and a nontender, often enlarged thyroid gland. The condition's usual course was a progression from hyperthyroidism to hypothyroidism, followed by a return to good health in two to six months once the thyroid inflammation subsided and the gland began to manufacture thyroid hormones again.

The accumulated evidence suggests that silent thyroiditis

may be the same condition as postpartum thyroiditis, brought on by factors other than pregnancy in the same susceptible population of men and women who have the inherited tendency to develop autoimmune thyroiditis.

Treatment of silent thyroiditis is the same as that used to counter postpartum thyroiditis. Usually patients require only symptomatic therapy, such as a beta-adrenergic blocking drug like propranolol, atenolol, or metoprolol in the early hyperthyroid phase of the illness. Rarely, for severe hyperthyroidism, a physician may recommend a steroid medication such as prednisone to reduce the inflammation within the thyroid and thus shorten the duration of the thyrotoxic state. Treatment with thyroid hormone is often needed during the later hypothyroid phase of the illness. For those individuals who remain hypothyroid, lifelong treatment will be required.

SUBACUTE THYROIDITIS, DEQUERVAIN'S DISEASE, GRANULOMATOUS THYROIDITIS

Subacute thyroiditis often follows an upper respiratory viral infection. Many different viruses have been linked to this condition, including those that cause mumps and measles, as well as some of those that cause the common cold. However, no one single virus has ever been identified as the specific cause of subacute thyroiditis. Since few people who develop a viral infection ever have evidence of thyroid inflammation, subacute thyroiditis is a relatively rare condition.

Typically the symptoms of subacute thyroiditis begin about two weeks after the first signs of a viral illness. When they start, you will probably look and feel as though you have an infection, with a painful enlarged thyroid, fever, muscle aches, and fatigue. An astute patient may notice that it is the *thyroid* that hurts in subacute thyroiditis, rather than the *inside* of the throat, as is the case with most sore throats. Because the thyroid pain seems to spread toward your jaw or ears, you may think you have a bad tooth or ear infection.

The history of a recent viral illness, followed by fever and an enlarged, tender thyroid, should make your physician suspect subacute thyroiditis. A high red blood cell sedimentation rate, indicating the presence of an inflammatory condition, is important evidence that the diagnosis is correct and helps differentiate this disorder from silent thyroiditis, which is not painful. In the test for sedimentation rate we measure how fast red blood cells settle in a narrow test tube. If you have an inflammatory condition such as this form of thyroiditis, the red blood cells usually settle faster than normal.

Like silent thyroiditis, this disorder follows a pattern of hyperthyroidism followed by hypothyroidism once the thyroid inflammation has subsided. The two lobes of the thyroid may be involved together or at different times, but in either instance the condition rarely lasts longer than twelve weeks. Fortunately this disorder is self-limited and usually responds readily to medical treatment. Since you may have a variety of symptoms, several types of treatment may be required. Your fever and thyroid pain can usually be controlled by aspirin alone. If you neck is very uncomfortable, your physician may recommend a more potent *nonsteroidal anti-inflammatory drug*, such as ibuprofen. On very rare occasions the pain may be so intense that the inflammation must be treated with a steroid medication such as cortisone or prednisone. The changing level of thyroid hormone in your blood may also require treatment. As with silent thyroiditis, during the early hyperthyroid phase of the disease, a beta-adrenergic blocking drug such as atenolol or propranolol is sometimes prescribed to decrease the effect of too much thyroid hormone on your body. Weeks later, if the thyroid-hormone level falls below normal, supplementary thyroxine (T4) tablets may be prescribed until your own thyroid begins working again. Ultimately you can expect total and complete recovery within five to six months.

ACUTE SUPPURATIVE THYROIDITIS

This is most often a disease of children but may occur at any age. If you develop this uncommon condition, you will be very sick. A bacterial infection is the usual cause of acute suppurative thyroiditis, so you will probably have chills, a very high fever, and a hot, tender thyroid; often there is an abscess within the gland.

As with other bacterial infections, antibiotics are required for treatment, and local surgical drainage or removal of abscessed tissue may be needed. In spite of the severity of acute suppurative thyroiditis, complete recovery is the usual outcome in this disease.

SUMMARY

Although the various forms of thyroiditis all involve inflammation of the thyroid gland, they are quite different disorders. Nevertheless they can all be readily diagnosed, and they all improve rapidly with the very effective treatments that are available.

SUBACUTE THYROIDITIS
by M. F.

I have been in general good health all my life. I work doing market research and have always had normal energy. As far as I know, neither I nor any other member of my family has ever had a thyroid problem.

I remember that I was feeling well until I got what seemed to be a cold. My throat felt sore and scratchy, but the difference this time was a swelling that appeared in the left side of my neck. I became extremely weak, even in the morning when I first got up. There were days when I seemed to have the strength to do some work and light housekeeping, but there were other days when I wanted just to stay in bed. I remember most the throbbing at the bottom of my neck on the left side with pain aching in my left ear at the same time. I felt so sick, I saw my doctor, who felt that I might have a strep throat and started treatment with penicillin and aspirin. I felt better within a day, and so well that in four days I stopped the aspirin and continued the penicillin. Much to my surprise I got sick again within a day with a recurrence of my sore throat, swollen neck, and extreme weakness. By this time I was also beginning to notice that my heart was racing. Sometimes it seemed to skip very fast for several minutes and then suddenly it would stop racing and beat normally again.

I called my doctor, who increased the penicillin. Aspirin was added again, and I soon felt better. Once again, however, when I stopped the aspirin after I felt better, all my symptoms returned.

I saw a thyroid specialist a few days later, and he diagnosed my condition as subacute thyroiditis. He explained that the aspirin was the main drug that was helping me and that there was no sign of any other infection at that time. Aspirin was restarted, and within a day my sore throat began to feel better, my strength began to return, and I felt generally improved. I stopped taking the penicillin.

Unfortunately the fast pulse continued, and when the doctor called me to say that my thyroid blood level was high, he also said that was what was causing my heart to race. I was glad that he understood the problem. I took a drug called propranolol four times a day, which slowed the heart rate but which, I understand, did not change the thyroid at all. For about a month and a half I took both aspirin and propranolol and felt fairly well, though not completely cured. During this time, interestingly, the soreness and swelling in my neck moved to the right side, while the left side of my neck became more normal. After about two months my thyroid level dropped, and I began to feel sluggish and cold and had some leg cramps too. My doctor prescribed thyroid-hormone tablets at that time, which raised my thyroid level to normal and returned me to good health. I stopped the thyroid pills after a month because by that time my thyroid had completely healed itself, and after that I felt normal without any medicine at all.

If I could give advice to other patients with this condition, I would say that aspirin seems to help a lot. If your doctor says you need propranolol, take it regularly, too, since each pill only works for a short time. Third, since the thyroid-hormone levels changed in my condition, they may change in yours. Check with your doctor as often as the doctor feels necessary until you are well. Fourth, be relieved that you have a condition that should go away completely and leave you with a normal thyroid gland and good health.

CHAPTER EIGHT

What About Your Family?

Graves' disease and Hashimoto's disease are inherited conditions, and your tendency to have either disorder was given to you in genes from your mother or your father. That parent, and some other relatives on that side of your family, may have already had an overactive or underactive thyroid like yours. On the other hand they may not be aware of any thyroid problem in the past or at present. But those relatives who share your genetic tendency toward Graves' disease may have an unrecognized thyroid abnormality, which you can help discover.

If your younger relatives with the inherited tendency to thyroid dysfunction have a thyroid problem, it is likely to be an overactive gland. Usually they are not hard to recognize, for their complaints will be fairly obvious and will include symptoms you have had yourself, such as nervousness, palpitations, shaky hands, weight loss, and perhaps prominent eyes as well. On the other hand, other relatives—especially those over the age of fifty, such as your parents and grandparents—may have hypothyroidism. Since symptoms of hypothyroidism may be mild (feeling cold, tired, a lack of energy, etc.), these older relatives may just accept those symptoms as signs of "getting old." Instead, if their symptoms are due to thyroid failure, they would feel better and be healthier if they were given treatment with thyroid hormone. Their thyroids may be failing for two reasons. First they may have had unrecognized hyperthyroidism in earlier years and may now be progressing to hypothyroidism in the natural course of their disease. On the other hand their thyroid glands may be failing because of Hashimoto's disease—chronic lymphocytic thyroiditis.

New observations suggest another important way to help

some of the women in your family who have inherited the tendency toward thyroid problems. These women are at high risk for thyroid dysfunction after pregnancy, so it would be helpful for them to tell their obstetricians and family doctors about the family predisposition to thyroid trouble. They should be examined and have a TSH blood test in the months after delivery to minimize the likelihood of letting thyroid dysfunction go unrecognized. As we will see in Chapter 13, the obstetrician may order a blood test for antithyroid antibodies during pregnancy to identify which women are at risk for postpartum thyroid problems and to find out whether there is a risk for thyroid dysfunction in their babies.

There is another side of this too. You and all of your relatives with this inherited tendency to thyroid trouble also have a greater-than-normal chance of developing certain other conditions. As described in more detail in Chapter 9, these involve many different parts of your body, and include the following:

- Hair: Prematurely gray—anyone who finds a gray hair before the age of thirty is considered "prematurely gray."
  Patchy hair loss *(alopecia areata)*—often mild and temporary, but may be extensive and long-lasting. It usually appears on the scalp but may involve other hairy areas, such as the beard.

- Skin: White patches on the skin *(vitiligo)*—white areas that are painless and often placed symmetrically in areas such as the knuckles, wrists, elbows, and neck.

- Blood: Anemia (a decrease in red blood cells) due to a lack of vitamin B12 *(pernicious anemia)* and not any of the anemias due to other causes.

- Joints: *Rheumatoid arthritis*—usually a symmetrical, deforming arthritis involving especially the hands, wrists, and feet. Morning stiffness is a common complaint.

- Eyes: Protrusion of the eyes *(exophthalmos)*. If the condition is mild, elevation of the eyelids may be all that is noted.

- Metabolism: *Diabetes mellitus* ("sugar diabetes"), which usually starts at a young age and requires insulin treatment.

We are not trying to imply that everyone who has diabetes or turns prematurely gray will have a thyroid problem. Rather we are saying that these disorders tend to occur in patients with Graves' disease and Hashimoto's disease, and in their relatives, with greater frequency than in the general population. The implications of this observation are twofold. First, physicians will tend to watch you and your family more carefully for the development of one of these problems that may require treatment. Pernicious anemia is such a condition—though at first it may be controlled by taking daily B12 tablets, ultimately a monthly injection of vitamin B12 is usually required (see Chapter 9). Second, some of these conditions are more obvious than hypothyroidism, and their presence can help you and your physician know which of your older relatives should be tested for that thyroid problem. Not everyone in your family should be tested, for that would be a waste of time and money for a lot of your relatives. But we can, and probably should, encourage those that are at greatest risk for a thyroid problem to see their family physician.

A search for thyroid and related conditions among the family of a young woman who has Graves' disease is shown in the hypothetical family tree in this chapter (see Figure 26).

The inheritance of thyroid disease in this family appears to have come from the mother's father down through the mother to the patient. Therefore the patient's maternal aunts and uncles should be evaluated for a thyroid condition, since they all have received half their genes from their hypothyroid father. The uncle with vitiligo and a goiter and the aunt with diabetes are perhaps more likely to develop hypothyroidism in later years than is the patient's apparently healthy aunt who has no signs of thyroid disease or a related condition. The patient's mother is "at risk" for a thyroid problem not only because of her prematurely gray hair but also because she has a hyperthyroid daughter.

Some of the hyperthyroid patient's brothers and sisters and one of her children are already showing signs that they have inherited a tendency toward thyroid disease, but only one sister has actually developed a problem (hyperthyroidism) requiring treatment.

WHO SHOULD BE TESTED?

Since *hypo*thyroidism tends to be a disease that comes on in later years, we tend to look for that condition only in those relatives who are over the age of fifty and who are on the side of the family that the thyroid tendency came from. In the example, that would be the maternal side. We would test them whether they looked and felt sick or not, since hypothyroidism is hard to recognize in many patients, especially if the condition is mild. If younger relatives looked or felt hypothyroid, they could be tested by their physicians, too, but we would not recommend this study if they felt well.

Similarly not everyone need be tested for *hyper*thyroidism on the mother's side in our hypothetical family. When that condition occurs, it is usually fairly obvious, and we could limit testing to younger or older relatives who have hyperactivity, rapid pulse, or other evidence suggestive of excessive thyroid function.

As noted above, we would also suggest screening women at risk for thyroid dysfunction if they become pregnant.

With that perspective in mind, if you or any of your relatives have a thyroid or related problem, you can examine your family to see if you can tell who should be checked for hypothyroidism or hyperthyroidism. In carrying out the evaluation of your family, you will probably find that several relatives on one side of the family will have had either a thyroid disorder or a thyroid-associated condition. In contrast those relatives on the other side of the family will probably have had few, if any, of the disorders. Figure 27 is a scheme that we have worked out that can help you trace various thyroid and related conditions through your family tree.

We would recommend that everyone over the age of fifty on the "thyroid side" of your family be examined by their physician for evidence of hypothyroidism. Below the age of fifty, only those relatives who feel sluggish and "run-down" need to be tested for hypothyroidism. Finally, relatives who seem hyperactive (fast pulse, increased sweating, nervousness, etc.) can be examined by their physicians for evidence of hyperthyroidism.

SCREENING FOR THYROID DISEASE (THE TSH TEST)

In addition to a medical examination, a simple test is available that can tell whether someone is hypothyroid or hyperthyroid. A single blood sample, taken at any time of the day, can be analyzed for thyroid-stimulating hormone (TSH). Hypothyroidism is associated with increased blood levels of TSH, while TSH is low or absent in patients with hyperthyroidism.

HOW SERIOUS ARE THESE CONDITIONS?

As we focus attention on the inheritance of thyroid disease within a family, we risk alarming patients needlessly about possible illnesses in their parents and children. Actually thyroid troubles rarely cause serious or life-threatening problems. A person who is hypothyroid can have mild hypothyroidism for years with no symptoms except perhaps mild fatigue. Similarly someone who is hyperthyroid can look and feel perfectly well (though perhaps somewhat hyperenergetic).

We are calling attention to these patterns of inheritance in an effort to find patients with mild conditions and thus improve their quality of life. For example an older person with hypothyroidism may well have more energy and productivity if his or her low thyroid levels are increased. And a young person with mild hyperthyroidism will usually feel

A Typical

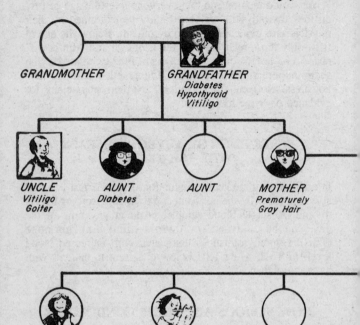

Figure 26 Affected members in a hypothetical family tree of a female patient.

Family Search

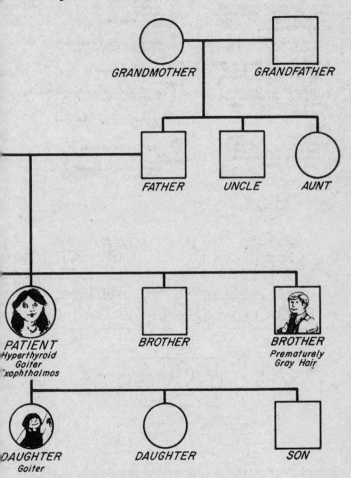

DIRECTIONS:

O = FEMALE   ☐ = MALE

THE DIAGRAM BELOW REPRESENTS YOUR
FAMILY TREE, AND WILL HELP YOU FIND
OUT WHO IN YOUR FAMILY IS "AT RISK"
FOR A THYROID DISORDER.

1. WRITE THE AGE OF EACH LIVING
   RELATIVE IN THE O OR ☐ BELOW.

2. FOR RELATIVES WHO HAVE DIED, WRITE
   THEIR AGE AT DEATH IN THE O OR ☐
   AND ADD A (†) AFTER THE NUMBER.

3. FOR RELATIVES WHO HAVE HAD ONE
   OR MORE OF THESE DISEASES, WRITE
   THE APPROPRIATE SYMBOL UNDER
   THE O OR ☐.

EXAMPLE:

A WOMAN WHO DIED AT AGE 65
AND HAD VITILIGO AND DIABETES,
AND BEGAN TO NOTICE GRAY
HAIR BEFORE AGE 30 WOULD BE
SHOWN AS FOLLOWS:

vitiligo
diabetes
premature gray hair

THYROID AND ASSOCIATED CONDITIONS

THYROID:
   overactive
   underactive
   thyroiditis
   goiter (enlarged thyroid)

HAIR:
   prematurely gray (any gray before age 30)
   alopecia areata (patchy hair loss)

SKIN:
   vitiligo (white skin spots)

BLOOD:
   pernicious anemia (anemia due to lack of Vitamin B_{12}
   and NOT other kinds of anemia)

JOINTS:
   rheumatoid arthritis (and NOT other forms
   of arthritis)

EYES:
   exophthalmos (protruding eyes)

METABOLISM:
   diabetes mellitus ("sugar diabetes") which requires
   insulin treatment

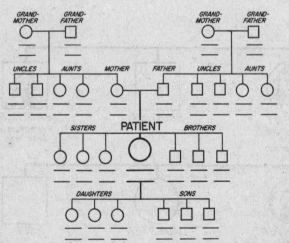

Figure 27 A scheme to help you trace your own family tree for
thyroid and related conditions.

calmer and be physically stronger if that condition is controlled.

In another way a search for disease might help an older relative on the "thyroid side" of your family, if he or she were discovered to have pernicious anemia. This condition, like hypothyroidism, can come on so slowly that it can remain unrecognized, yet cause sluggishness due to the anemia (low blood count) or clumsiness and loss of balance due to involvement of the nervous system. It is the authors' custom to test for pernicious anemia by means of a blood test for vitamin B12 in patients over the age of sixty who have had Graves' or Hashimoto's disease, or who are on the "thyroid side" of such a family. A full discussion of pernicious anemia (as well as the other conditions that are associated with Graves' disease and Hashimoto's disease) can be found in Chapter 9.

WHAT WILL THE TREATMENT BE?

When identified, an underactive thyroid is usually treated by the patient's physician with small amounts of thyroid-hormone supplementation given as a thyroxine tablet to be taken once a day. Starting doses in those individuals over fifty years of age must be small, since some older persons do not tolerate sudden big changes in their thyroid-hormone levels. Thereafter the dose is increased every month or so until the T4 and TSH are normal.

Since the symptoms of hyperthyroidism are due to the presence of too much thyroid hormone in the body, treatment of that condition is aimed at reducing the production of hormone by the thyroid gland. This can be done by medicines that affect the thyroid. Alternatively it is possible to decrease the production of thyroid hormone either by removing part of the gland in an operation or by destroying some of the thyroid tissue with radioactive iodine. In practice, treatment is individualized by physicians, and depends upon each patient's particular circumstances, including age and other health problems.

SUMMARY

We have prepared this guide as part of an ongoing effort to reach people who need treatment for thyroid disease and to educate them about their disorder. We hope that you decide to carry out this thyroid search within your family and that you will let your family physician know the results. Your physician should be able to aide you if you have questions about how to do the search or about which relatives should be tested for thyroid problems.

CHAPTER NINE

Graves' Disease, Hashimoto's Thyroiditis, and Some Related Conditions: *Addison's Disease, Allergy, Pernicious Anemia, Rheumatoid Arthritis, Diabetes, Dyslexia, and Disorders of the Eyes, Emotions, Hair, Heart, Liver, Muscles, Nerves, and Skin*

> For a long period I had from time to time met with a very remarkable form of general anaemia, occurring without any discoverable cause whatever.... The leading and characteristic features of the morbid state to which I would direct attention are, anaemia, general languor and debility, remarkable feebleness of the heart's action, irritability of the stomach, and a peculiar change of colour in the skin, occurring in connection with a diseased condition of the "suprarenal capsules."
>
> —Thomas Addison (1855)

Thomas Addison believed that he was describing the features of a disease caused by failure of two glands located above the kidneys, now known as the *adrenal glands*, which make *cortisone* and other steroid hormones. Actually his descriptions suggest that, in addition to adrenal failure, some of his patients also had *pernicious anemia*, a blood condition caused by a deficiency of vitamin B12. It is not surprising that some of Addison's patients had both diseases, for we now know that there is a slight tendency for the two conditions to occur together.

From time to time physicians have recognized similar relationships, in which diseases occur together more often than chance alone would allow. In 1926 M. B. Schmidt, a physician in Germany, described two patients in whom both the adrenal and thyroid glands had failed. Since then more than 125 patients with both disorders have been described, enough to make us realize that something more than an "accident of nature" makes this rare combination happen.

In several places in this book we have commented on the relationship between Graves' disease and Hashimoto's disease, which tend to occur in the same families, sometimes in the same patients, and which may even be different presentations of a single disease process. This chapter is about the other conditions that tend to occur in patients with Graves' disease and Hashimoto's disease, and in their relatives as well. Some, like the prominent eyes of Graves' disease known as *exophthalmos*, have been well studied, and their relationship to thyroid problems carefully examined. Others, such as some of the associated skin disorders, are less well understood in regard to their relationship to the thyroid.

This chapter is not about those bodily changes that occur due to high or low thyroid-hormone levels. High hormone levels, for example, can raise your upper eyelids, make your skin soft and smooth, and cause your hair to become fine and delicate. The high hormone levels do not, however, cause your eyes to protrude, make white patches of *vitiligo* appear on your skin, or produce the patchy baldness we call *alopecia areata*. The latter problems are diseases in their own right and are the subject of this chapter.

These are not, in general, serious problems about which thyroid patients should be concerned. Many, such as *alopecia areata*, are not helped much by treatment, but tend to go away after a period of time. Others, such as *pernicious anemia* or vitiligo, can be cured or controlled by appropriate treatment. Some, such as *Addison's disease*, are so uncommon that even thyroid specialists rarely see a patient with this condition. Nevertheless we believe there should be a place in this book to which patients with Graves' disease or Hashimoto's disease could refer if they discover that they or one of their relatives has one of these problems.

DISORDERS OF OTHER ENDOCRINE GLANDS—
ADRENAL, OVARY, PARATHYROID AND PITUITARY

Your thyroid is one of many endocrine glands, and autoimmune inflammations like that occurring in Hashimoto's thyroiditis may occur in those other glands too. When the inflammation leads to scarring and tissue damage, the glands may fail to produce enough hormones for your needs. The symptoms that result depend on the function of those hormones.

Your adrenal glands make *cortisone* and other *steroid hormones*, which are released into your blood stream daily and are especially important in your response to stressful situations. Adrenal failure is an uncommon condition, occurring in only one individual per 100,000 of the population. In most patients with Addison's disease, glandular damage is due to an immune attack on the tissues of the adrenal glands. If your adrenal glands fail, you will experience fatigue, loss of energy, weakness, and darkening of your skin, especially over your joints and inside your mouth. This condition is treated by replacing the hormones that the adrenals no longer make in sufficient amounts (cortisone and related steroid hormones).

Some women suffer from *oophoritis*, a painless autoimmune inflammation of their ovaries. In this condition antibodies to ovarian tissue may be found in the bloodstream, and inflammation and scarring have been demonstrated in the ovarian tissues of affected individuals. Though rare, oophoritis is a condition your physician will consider if a woman experiences early menopause.

Autoimmune damage to your parathyroid glands may lead to calcium deficiency (hypocalcemia). Symptoms of this condition include mood changes, numbness, and tingling around the mouth and in the fingers and toes, muscle cramps, and, very rarely, convulsive seizures. Though associated with autoimmune disorders, it is actually a very rare cause of low calcium levels among thyroid patients. The more common cause of hypocalcemia is accidental damage to the parathyroid glands after thyroid surgery. If you develop hypoparathyroidism, your physician will likely prescribe calcium and vitamin D tablets to eliminate your symptoms by adjusting your doses of these medications to bring your calcium into the normal range.

Even the pituitary, the master gland of the endocrine system, may suffer immune damage. This rare disorder (termed *hypophysitis* because *hypophysis* is another name for the pituitary) occurs most often in women during or just after pregnancy. In the thirty patients described in one report, slightly more than half experienced headaches, 32 percent lost part of their vision (the pituitary is located very near the optic nerves), and most experienced fatigue and weakness as other glands, such as the adrenals and the thyroid, which depend on the pituitary for stimulation, began to fail. Treatment involves replacing the hormones that are lost when pituitary function declines.

ALLERGY

Medical studies done many years ago suggested that some allergic disorders seemed to occur with increased frequency among patients with thyroid problems. Unfortunately this is an area that has received little study during recent years when thyroid tests have become accurate and specific. Therefore it is not possible to say whether these conditions are indeed more common in patients with thyroid problems than in the general population. Some patients who have or who have had thyroid problems seem to have a greater-than-normal tendency to develop *hives* from time to time. These red, itchy welts on the skin do not necessarily come at times when the thyroid is malfunctioning. They generally respond to treatment with antihistamine drugs.

ANEMIA AND OTHER BLOOD DISORDERS

Anemia is a disorder characterized by a decrease in the number of red blood cells that carry oxygen to various body tissues. If you have hypothyroidism, you may also have an associated mild anemia as one manifestation of the general slowing of your body functions that occurs in your condition. The anemia usually causes no symptoms and corrects itself when your hypothyroidism is treated. It is not a separate disease, but is due instead to the low thyroid-hormone level.

A more serious type of anemia, known as *pernicious anemia*, is a separate disease that tends to occur in older patients and their relatives who have or have had Graves' disease or Hashimoto's thyroiditis. This kind of anemia is caused by a deficiency of vitamin B12. Under normal circumstances cells lining your stomach make a substance known as *intrinsic factor* that enables your body to absorb vitamin B12 from food. Some individuals lose the ability to absorb vitamin B12, due to failure of the cells that make intrinsic factor. The damage seems to be caused by a self-destructive process involving the body's immune system, similar to what occurs in Addison's and Hashimoto's diseases. Vitamin B12 is an important ingredient in the manufacturing of red blood cells, and if levels of this vitamin fall, anemia may result. Vitamin B12 is also important in nourishing your nervous system, so if you develop pernicious anemia, you may also experience numbness and tingling of your hands and feet, loss of balance, and even leg weakness. It is not clear how many patients who have thyroid-function problems also develop pernicious anemia. Some studies have suggested that as many as 5 percent of patients with Graves' disease and 10 percent of those who have Hashimoto's disease may develop this condition. Since pernicious anemia tends to develop in later years, it is probably even more common in older patients with either condition.

It is the authors' custom to measure the blood level of vitamin B12 in every patient over the age of sixty who has ever had Graves' disease or Hashimoto's thyroiditis. We do this because pernicious anemia is both common and treatable. If your blood level of vitamin B12 appears low or borderline low, another test, known as a *Schilling test*, can be performed. This test demonstrates whether you have difficulty absorbing vitamin B12 from your food. If you do have pernicious anemia, it can be easily treated. On the basis of new research your physician may choose to treat you initially with tablets of B12 to see if you are able to absorb enough of the vitamin to restore your blood level to normal and thus cure the condition. However, since your body's ability to absorb B12 tends to decrease with time, you will probably need treatment with a monthly intramuscular injection of vitamin B12 as you grow older.

Platelet disorders are also more common in this group of thyroid patients than they are in the general population. Normally you have about 2.5 million platelets in every teaspoonful of your blood. Despite their small size, they play a major role in helping your blood to clot normally. Some thyroid patients experience easy bruising due to a decrease in the number or function of their platelets. The bruising can become much worse if you take aspirin, or one of the *nonsteroidal anti-inflammatory drugs*, such as ibuprofen (Advil or Motrin) or Naprosyn. If that is your situation, your physician may choose to order a platelet count or check your platelet function with a "bleeding time" test, which tells how long it takes your blood to clot. He or she may also recommend that you take an alternative pain medication such as acetaminophen (Tylenol), which will not worsen your bleeding tendency.

Very rarely immune processes may destroy large numbers of platelets, producing *thrombocytopenic purpura.* The word *purpura* refers to the red or blue bruises that appear on the skin in this condition, especially on the legs. Tiny purplish-red spots known as *petechiae* that represent smaller areas of bleeding within the skin are also commonly present in this condition. If you develop this type of rash, your physician is likely to consider it an emergency and order an immediate platelet count because of the risk of more serious bleeding elsewhere. If thrombocytopenic purpura proves to be your problem, treatment is usually helpful, and often includes steroid medication.

ARTHRITIS

Some patients with Graves' or Hashimoto's disease also have a tendency to certain kinds of tendon and joint inflammation. Painful *tendonitis* and *bursitis* of the shoulder, for example, was reported in 6.7 percent of patients but occurs in only about 1.7 percent of the general population.

Rheumatoid arthritis is a more serious disease, in which there is a symmetrical inflammation of many joints of the body, most typically the knuckles, wrists, and elbows. It is also characterized by joint stiffness that is most severe in the morning. Severe rheumatoid arthritis appears to be only slightly more common among patients with thyroid dysfunction than in the general population. If you have hyper- or hypothyroidism, you may notice mild morning joint pain and stiffness. If so, like patients with rheumatoid arthritis, you can benefit from treatment with heat, aspirin, and related drugs. On the other hand, some hypothyroid patients have joint pain and stiffness that improves when they are treated with thyroid medication.

DIABETES MELLITUS

Among patients with Graves' or Hashimoto's diseases and their relatives, there is an increased incidence of the type of diabetes that usually begins in children or young adults and needs to be treated with insulin (so-called *juvenile-onset diabetes*). Although both are due to self-destructive immune processes that damage the thyroid and the pancreas respectively, the two disorders do not usually occur in the same individuals. However, if you do have both conditions at once, an overactive thyroid will often make your diabetes more severe and more difficult to control with insulin. Treatment of your thyroid problem, in that case, should make your diabetes easier to control.

DYSLEXIA

On the basis of recent research, it is evident that learning disabilities *(dyslexia)* are more common in families in which someone has had hyperthyroidism or Hashimoto's disease than in the general population.

Children with dyslexia may have a variety of problems, including delays in physical or speech development, poor spelling or handwriting, stuttering, right-left confusion, and reversals of numbers or letters. They may be good at math and have better-than-average verbal skills, and are often especially gifted in other ways, including athletics, art, and music. On the other hand they may have real difficulty reading and paying attention in class. Therefore, though these children are usually very bright, poor academic performance is not uncommon and may lead to loss of self-esteem. The condition occurs more commonly in males than in females, and affected children are often left-handed or ambidextrous.

Therefore if you or someone in your family has thyroid dysfunction or chronic thyroiditis and there are children in the family with these sorts of learning and/or attention problems, you would do well to have them checked by a specialist in learning disabilities, who should be available through your school or family physician.

Dyslexia is treatable anytime—the earlier the better—and the academic improvement in special-help programs may be striking. Remember that the learning disabilities are not caused by thyroid problems and in fact are usually more evident in males, while the related thyroid troubles tend to occur in the females in the family.

EYE ENLARGEMENT AND INFLAMMATION

Elevation of the upper eyelids may occur in anyone with hyperthyroidism from any cause, anytime the blood level of thyroid hormone is above normal. For example patients who are hyperthyroid because of too much thyroid-hormone medication may have raised upper eyelids causing their eyes to appear enlarged or staring. In this situation, however, the eyes do not actually protrude.

If you have Graves' disease, you may develop protrusion and inflammation of your eyes without there being any evidence of infection. It is likely to begin about the time your thyroid becomes overactive, but it may precede your hyperthyroidism or occur years after your thyroid function has become normal. Very rarely the eye disorder may occur without your having any obvious abnormality of thyroid function at any time in your life.

More serious eye problems may occur in patients with Graves' disease and (less commonly) Hashimoto's thyroiditis. The severity of these conditions is unrelated to the blood level of thyroid hormone. If the condition is mild, you may have only redness and irritation of your eyes. On the other hand in those rare instances when the inflammation is more severe, your eyes may protrude, you may have double vision, and your sight may be threatened.

It should be pointed out that thyroid eye disease does not necessarily progress in an orderly fashion from mild to severe in any given patient. In fact a rapid decrease in vision can occur due to pressure upon the optic nerve in a patient with only minimal swelling of the eyelids. For this reason, if you have Graves' disease and begin to show signs of eye trouble, you should have a complete eye examination. If your eye involvement is severe, your physician may refer you to an *ophthalmologist* (eye specialist), who will have at his or her disposal all of the equipment needed to evaluate the various eye problems that may occur in Graves' disease. Your vision can be accurately tested. The amount of eye protrusion can be accurately measured with an *exophthalmometer*. The cornea and other tissues of your eye can be examined by the use of a microscopelike instrument known as a *slit lamp*. *Ultrasound* pictures of your eye and eye socket *(orbit)* may be taken, using sound waves in a technique similar to radar. Alternatively your physician may request special X rays of your orbits done by *computerized tomography (CT scan)*, or by a newer technique called *magnetic resonance imaging (MRI)*. These techniques will provide a clear picture of the inflamed tissues behind your eye.

Treatment of your eye condition will depend upon the kind of eye disease you have and whether it is getting worse. Mild inflammation may be treated simply by elevating the head of your bed at night and by lubricating your eyes with drops of "artificial tears." On the other hand, if you have a severe and rapidly progressive inflammatory condition with double vision or decreased vision, you may require special glasses or treatment with steroids. If your eye tissues continue to swell despite the use of steroid hormones, additional therapy is available. This may include X-ray treatments to the tissues behind the eye or surgery on the bony orbit *(surgical decompression)* to relieve the increased pressure behind your eye.

Fortunately serious eye problems are rare among thyroid patients. When they do occur, the treatment methods are excellent and are usually successful in improving the problem. Occasionally excessive drooping of the upper or lower eyelids may cause cosmetic problems, but plastic eye surgery can be very helpful for such patients.

HAIR LOSS AND PREMATURELY GRAY HAIR

Changes in thyroid function are associated with a change in the body's use of oxygen (metabolic rate). If the metabolic rate is too high or too low, hair growth may be imperfect. As a result, you may lose some of your hair if your thyroid is either overactive or underactive from any cause. In most cases your hair loss will be generalized and mild, and your hair growth will return to normal as soon as your thyroid problem is controlled.

Occasionally, patients with Graves' or Hashimoto's disease or their relatives may notice a patchy hair loss instead. This condition, known as *alopecia areata*, is characterized by bald spots anywhere on the body where hair grows, including your scalp and beard. Generally the condition goes away by itself after several months, regardless of the level of thyroid function and thyroid treatment, but occasionally such hair loss is permanent.

Physicians have recognized for some time that prematurely gray hair, by which we mean hair that starts to become gray before age thirty, occurs more frequently in patients with thyroid dysfunction than in the general population. This common and easily recognized condition is of course harmless, but it is important because it can be helpful to you in tracing the pattern of inheritance of thyroid diseases within your family (see Chapter 8).

HEART TROUBLE: ATRIAL FIBRILLATION AND MITRAL VALVE PROLAPSE

On May 7, 1991, President George Bush was jogging when his heart suddenly began to beat in a rapid and erratic manner. He had developed *atrial fibrillation*, a common rhythm disturbance in older people with underlying heart problems, such as coronary disease or trouble with one of the heart valves. But the President was not known to have these problems and seemed fit.

Mr. Bush's physicians also knew that atrial fibrillation is a common complication of hyperthyroidism, and immediately ordered appropriate tests, which led to the diagnosis of Graves' disease. As often happens, control of the President's hyperthyroidism helped normalize his heart rhythm.

Today physicians test for hyperthyroidism in anyone who develops atrial fibrillation, especially older individuals who may have very few other manifestations of thyroid overactivity (see Chapter 14). In one research study atrial fibrillation was found in 25 percent of individuals who had developed hyperthyroidism over the age of sixty. In another report 28 percent of patients with such mild hyperthyroidism that their thyroid-hormone levels were normal and whose only abnormal blood test was a low TSH level developed atrial fibrillation over a ten year period.

If you have atrial fibrillation and hyperthyroidism, control of your thyroid problem may restore normal heart rhythm. You have about a 50 percent chance of this happening if you are younger than fifty, and 25 percent if you are over sixty. If your heart rhythm fails to become normal with treatment, or if you have atrial fibrillation and no thyroid problem is found, treatment with heart medications and anticoagulants is usually recommended to prevent the formation of blood clots in your fibrillating heart. Otherwise such clots could escape from the heart and cause a stroke if carried through your bloodstream to your brain.

So if you or anyone you know develops atrial fibrillation, expect the involved physician to look for hyperthyroidism with measurements of thyroid hormone levels and a TSH blood test.

Your *mitral heart valve* is located in the left side of your heart between your left atrium (which collects blood from your lungs) and your left ventricle (which pumps blood out to your body). Between 5 and 10 percent of the general population have a deformed mitral heart valve, which doesn't close properly and may leak. A physician listening to your heart may suspect this condition (known as *mitral valve prolapse*) if he or she hears a characteristic extra "click" sound and/or a murmur. If you have this problem, you may occasionally experience various types of chest pains or palpitations, though the condition is rarely life-threatening.

Mitral valve prolapse has been reported to be unusually common among patients with autoimmune thyroid disease. In studies done in the late 1980s, sensitive heart examinations known as *echocardiograms* performed on thyroid patients suggested that 41 percent of those with Hashimoto's thyroiditis and 43 percent of those with active or treated Graves' disease had mitral valve prolapse. Such a high reported incidence of this heart problem concerned many physicians and thyroid patients. However, in recent years improvements in ultrasound technique and interpretation have led other investigators to suggest that the true incidence of mitral valve prolapse is probably much lower than originally suggested, but possibly still higher than in the general population.

There are various degrees of severity of mitral valve prolapse, and many patients have no symptoms and need no treatment. On the other hand, if your physician hears a murmur due to valve leakage or an echocardiogram shows significant valve distortion, your doctor may recommend antibiotics to protect your valve from infection at times of dental work, surgery, or infections.

INTESTINAL DISORDERS

Inflammatory bowel disease is a general term which includes *regional enteritis (Crohn's disease)* and *ulcerative colitis*. Both conditions seem to be caused by inflammation and scarring due to immune processes such as those that damage thyroid cells in thyroiditis. Patients with either condition may experience repeated episodes of crampy abdominal pain, fever, and diarrhea that may contain mucus and blood. Both conditions are slightly more common in families in which someone has had autoimmune thyroid disease.

Symptoms and treatment will vary according to the severity of the problem, but much can be learned by careful tests, which usually include blood tests, intestinal X rays, and examination and biopsy of the involved intestine. Fortunately both conditions are relatively uncommon, and a great deal can be accomplished through treatment that includes an improved diet, medication, and occasionally intestinal surgery.

LEFT-HANDEDNESS AND AMBIDEXTERITY

Left-handedness tends to be more common among men than women, while autoimmune thyroid disease tends to happen more in women. Thus if you try to find out the frequency of any degree of left-handedness among thyroid patients, the answer you get depends on whether you ask men or women with thyroid trouble about hand preference.

Two of the authors (DSC and LCW) asked seventy-four men with Graves' or Hashimoto's disease about this and found that twelve were pure left-handers, forty ambidextrous, and only twenty-two pure right-handers. Thus 70 percent of these men had some degree of left-handedness. In contrast among twenty-four individuals with other types of thyroid problems, such as benign and cancerous nodules, only two were left-handed and four ambidextrous for a total of 25 percent, 75 percent being right-handed.*

So if you or someone in your family is completely or partially left-handed, this may be a clue that there is also a tendency to autoimmune problems including Graves' and Hashimoto's diseases in your family.

*Wood LC, Cooper DS. Autoimmune thyroid disease, left-handedness, and developmental dyslexia. *Psychoneuroendocrinology*. 1992; 17: 95–99.

LIVER DISEASE AND JAUNDICE

Some patients with thyroid dysfunction have an associated tendency to develop *jaundice*, a yellow color of the skin caused by increased blood levels of a substance known as *bilirubin*. Though our knowledge of this relationship is incomplete, some of these patients with mild jaundice have a harmless condition known as *Gilbert's disease*. In these individuals jaundice develops from time to time because the liver does not clear bilirubin from the blood properly. Before this condition was understood, such patients were occasionally misdiagnosed as having hepatitis. Now, however, we have better tests available and can easily recognize this form of jaundice when it occurs.

Patients with autoimmune thyroid disease are at slightly increased risk for a more serious type of liver disease known as *primary biliary cirrhosis*. In this rare condition, jaundice and other evidence of liver failure develop when the bile ducts become blocked due to an autoimmune inflammatory process within the liver. In one group of ninety-five patients with primary biliary cirrhosis, 26 percent had evidence of antithyroid antibodies in their blood, and 16 percent showed evidence of thyroid failure ranging from an increased blood level of TSH to symptomatic hypothyroidism. So if you develop jaundice, your doctor may order tests to see if you have biliary cirrhosis. If that is your problem, your treatment will depend on your symptoms and the severity of your problem at the time the diagnosis is made.

LUPUS ERYTHEMATOSUS

Lupus erythematosus is a rare condition caused by immune inflammation in many tissues of the body. Arthritis, skin rashes (often induced by sunlight), and kidney, lung, and heart problems are common. In addition antibodies to thyroid tissue are frequently observed. In one report doctors found that among twenty-eight patients with lupus one was hyperthyroid, three hypothyroid, and an additional fourteen had antithyroid antibodies in their blood. Although lupus is extremely rare among thyroid patients, thyroid troubles appear to be fairly common among individuals who have lupus. So if you or someone in your family has lupus, your physician may look for thyroid trouble in family members.

NERVE AND MUSCLE PROBLEMS

"Painful hands and sleepless nights" are the reasons one neurologist says patients seek help for *carpal tunnel syndrome*. A major nerve, known as the median nerve, passes from your forearm to your palm through a very narrow space known as the carpal tunnel (from the Latin word *carpus*, which means "wrist"). Inflammation and swelling in this area (more common in thyroid patients than in the general population) may compress your median nerve—this may lead to burning, numbness, pain, and weakness in your thumb and adjacent three fingers. Once suspected, carpal tunnel syndrome can be confirmed by an *electromyogram*, or *EMG*, which tests the function of your median nerve. If the diagnosis is correct, your physician may recommend treatment with an anti-inflammatory drug such as aspirin, ibuprofen (Advil or Motrin), or Naprosyn. Your physician may also recommend a "cock-up splint" to immobilize the joint and prevent nighttime pain due to pressure on the nerve caused by unconscious flexing of the wrist while asleep. Steroid medications can be injected into the carpal tunnel itself. A final possibility is wrist surgery to enlarge the carpal tunnel; this course is usually considered if muscle function and hand sensation are threatened.

A rare muscle disease known as *myasthenia gravis* is about ten times as common in patients with Graves' disease as in the general population, where it affects about thirty-three people per million. If you develop this condition, you will feel weak, and the more work you try to do, the weaker your muscles will become. You may also have double vision and difficulty in swallowing. If you have hyperthyroidism, too, it should be promptly treated and your thyroid level brought to normal, for an abnormal hormone level may cause the muscular weakness to worsen.

Multiple sclerosis is a slow, intermittently progressive

disorder characterized by attacks of neurological disturbances, such as eye troubles (sudden double vision or temporary loss of color vision or all vision in one or both eyes), pain, weakness, tremors, or loss of balance. The symptoms of multiple sclerosis are caused by inflammation and scarring from autoimmune damage within the brain and other parts of the nervous system, like those in thyroid tissues of patients with chronic thyroiditis. Treatment can help but will depend on the nature and severity of the neurological events.

Periodic paralysis is an exceedingly uncommon condition characterized by episodes of sudden, complete, temporary paralysis, often occurring after exercise or after consumption of a meal containing a lot of carbohydrate (starch and sugar). A lowering of the blood level of potassium is sometimes associated with the period of paralysis, and in patients so afflicted, treatment with potassium may help to control the weakness. Some patients with periodic paralysis also have hyperthyroidism due to Graves' disease. If so, control of the thyroid problem usually brings an end to the attacks of paralysis. For some reason Asian patients seem to be more subject than others to develop periodic paralysis in association with hyperthyroidism.

PSYCHIATRIC PROBLEMS

Bipolar disease is a relatively new term that psychiatrists use to describe individuals whose emotions tend to swing from highs to lows, elation to the "blues," more than most other people. A subgroup of this population experience "rapid cycling," meaning that they have at least four major highs and lows per year. In studies of patients with rapid-cycling bipolar disease (85 percent of whom are women), 25 to 50 percent have been shown to have evidence of thyroid deficiency. Some feel well, and their only evidence of thyroid failure is an increased level of TSH in their blood. Others are clearly hypothyroid.

Physicians have also learned that lithium, a particularly effective drug in treating bipolar disease, may reduce thyroid function and cause hypothyroidism in susceptible individuals, primarily those with a tendency to autoimmune thyroid disorders. Therefore if you or someone in your family experiences these major mood swings, your physician may order tests for thyroid problems including a measurement of your blood level of TSH. If treatment with lithium is chosen, follow-up TSH blood tests from time to time are indicated. If your thyroid fails, you can continue lithium treatment and simply add thyroid hormone therapy to correct your thyroid deficiency.

Some physicians screen patients for a tendency to thyroid dysfunction by means of a blood test for antithyroid antibodies before they prescribe lithium treatment. It seems reasonable that those patients with a positive antibody test should have periodic TSH tests throughout the period of treatment with lithium. In reality most physicians order occasional TSH tests on any patient taking lithium.

SJÖGREN'S SYNDROME

In 1933 Swedish physician Henrik Sjögren described a group of women whose chronic arthritis was accompanied by dry eyes and a dry mouth. *Sjögren's syndrome* is an autoimmune condition caused by lymphocytic inflammation and scarring in tear and salivary glands as well as the mucous glands of the vagina.

If you experience frequent eye irritation, dry mouth, or excessive vaginal dryness, it is probably due to common problems such as hay fever or air pollution. But if your examination suggests Sjögren's syndrome, your physician can look for evidence of a more serious reduction in tearing with a *Shirmer test* in which the tip of a thin strip of absorbent paper is placed under your lower eyelid. Your physician can then estimate your ability to make tears by how wet the paper becomes in a fixed time. Alternatively a biopsy of tiny glands on the inner surface of your lip may be recommended to find out if you have this condition.

If you have this rare condition, your treatment will depend on the severity of your symptoms. Artificial tears and lubricating ointments may help. Occasionally steroid hormones are prescribed. More information and a lot of helpful advice can be obtained from the Sjögren's Foundation (see Appendix 7).

SKIN DISORDERS

If your thyroid is overactive from any cause, you will probably notice thinning of your skin and increased sweating. Conversely if your thyroid is underactive, your skin may become thick, rough, and dry. Your skin will return to normal gradually after treatment restores your thyroid hormone level to normal. These problems are due to thyroid dysfunction and are not separate diseases.

Pretibial myxedema is a very rare condition in which reddish, raised, firm, usually nontender lumps develop on the front of the legs and on top of the feet of a few patients with Graves' disease. It arises when substances known as *mucopolysaccharides* are deposited in these areas, but we still do not know why they appear and why only the legs and feet tend to be involved in most patients who have this condition. If you have this problem, it usually responds quite well to treatment with cortisone creams. For greatest effectiveness, these creams can be put on your skin at night under a plastic wrapping material, such as Saran Wrap, and held in place by paper adhesive tape.

Vitiligo is a thyroid-related condition in which milk-white patches appear where the skin has lost its normal pigment. It occurs in association with both Graves' disease and Hashimoto's disease and is generally unrelated to the state of the patient's thyroid activity. In most patients the white spots are small and therefore unnoticed, though in some patients vitiligo may be so extensive as to require dermatologic treatment. In recent years dermatologists have begun using drugs known as *psoralens*, which, when acted upon by sunlight, can increase the amount of skin pigment in most patients with vitiligo. This form of treatment is not for everybody, but if you have vitiligo and want the latest information about available treatments, you should ask your physician to recommend a good dermatologist for a consultation.

One of the most common skin-related symptoms that

thyroid patients report is itching. Some of this may be caused by dryness, but often a condition known as *dermatographism* may play a role in the itching. Simply stated, skin trauma such as scratching or even a hot shower produces hives that itch. This troublesome symptom can be helped by substituting lukewarm baths for hot showers and avoiding substances that irritate the skin (wool is a common culprit).

Scleroderma is a rare condition characterized by inflammation and scarring of the skin and many internal organs. Symptoms vary depending on which organs are most affected by this autoimmune disorder. Pain, swelling, and stiffness of the fingers and knees are common in this condition, which may also be accompanied by cold-induced blanching and pain in fingers and toes due to arterial constriction *(Raynaud's syndrome)*. One patient study found inflammation and scarring in the thyroid glands of 14 percent of seventy patients with scleroderma. In another study blood tests showed that seven of twenty-seven patients with scleroderma (26 percent) had hypothyroidism. Fortunately despite this association very few thyroid patients develop scleroderma.

Dermatitis herpetaformis is an extremely rare skin condition in which intensely itchy, fluid-filled blisters, reddish bumps, and hives tend to be symmetrically distributed over your limbs, buttocks, and back. If you develop this very uncommon condition, your physician will likely suggest that you consult a dermatologist to be certain of the diagnosis and for guidance in treatment. In one series of fifty patients with dermatitis herpetaformis, twenty-six were found to have thyroid dysfunction. Though it is rare among thyroid patients, if someone in your family has this skin problem, they should also be tested for thyroid trouble.

SUMMARY

In this chapter we have presented a spectrum of conditions that are autoimmune themselves or associated with thyroid autoimmune disorders. No one with either hyper- or hypothyroidism, Graves' disease or Hashimoto's disease, is likely to have more than one or two of these conditions. But we have described them in the hope that they will be recognized and treated if they do occur in a thyroid patient or close relative. When one of these problems is recognized in a relative, that individual's physician is likely to suggest thyroid testing to exclude an associated thyroid problem. Since a serum TSH test can diagnose either hyper- or hypothyroidism, such screening in an asymptomatic person may well be limited to that test alone, saving the unnecessary expense of a more elaborate thyroid evaluation.

CHAPTER TEN

Thyroid Lumps and Tumors

Nodules of the thyroid are common. Many are benign and only a few, malignant. It is difficult, however, to ferret out the few malignant lesions from the far more numerous benign nodules.

—From Wang CA, Vickery AL, and Maloof F,
Needle biopsy of the thyroid,
Surgery, Gynecology, and Obstetrics 1976; 143: 365–68.

Thyroid lumps, or nodules are fairly common problems in the general population. A careful thyroid examination will reveal thyroid lumps larger than a centimeter (½ inch) in diameter in about 4 percent of the population. Furthermore autopsy studies in which the entire gland has been carefully examined have shown that small thyroid nodules are in fact much more common than that and can be found in more than half the population.

Fortunately most of these nodules are harmless—few contain cancer, and most require no treatment. Although thyroid cancer does occur, it is an extremely rare condition. The United States Public Health Service reports that in one year only twenty-five people per million in the population will be found to have a cancer in the thyroid gland. Therefore if you or your physician have found a lump in your neck (Figure 28), don't panic. Although it is important that the nodule be evaluated, it is unlikely to be malignant. It is far more likely to be benign.

EVALUATING A THYROID NODULE

Your physician will take a careful medical history, examine your neck, and perform some laboratory tests to gain the information needed to decide if your thyroid lump needs medical or surgical therapy. As shown in Table 2, by talking with you about your medical history, your physician can

117

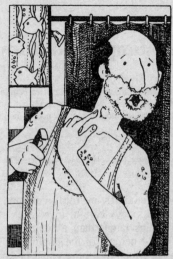

Figure 28 If you find a lump in your neck, see your doctor.

get information that can help determine whether your nodule is likely to be benign or cancerous. For example a lump is more likely to be benign if you are an adult woman who has symptoms of an overactive or underactive thyroid, or who has relatives with benign conditions, such as chronic lymphocytic thyroiditis or a goiter. On the other hand, if you have a family history of thyroid cancer, the nodule grew quickly, the nodule is associated with enlarged lymph glands, or if you had X-ray treatments to your face or neck sometime in the past, chances are higher that the lump is a cancer. There is also a greater likelihood of cancer if you have noticed a change in your voice, hoarseness, or trouble in swallowing (suggesting that a cancer is pressing against nearby parts of your neck).

During a physical examination your physician will feel your thyroid gland. Benign nodules tend to be soft and fleshy and are not associated with enlargement of nearby lymph glands. The rest of the thyroid may also feel abnormal. It is reassuring if more than one nodule can be felt within the thyroid, since this is an indication of a generalized thyroid disease, such as a nodular goiter. On the other hand, if your doctor feels a single, hard, fixed lump in an otherwise apparently normal gland, that nodule is more likely to contain cancer. The likelihood of cancer increases if the lump seems "fixed" to nearby structures within your neck or if it is associated with swelling of nearby lymph glands.

After your physician has examined your neck, tests should be recommended depending on the findings in your examination. Fortunately the testing techniques available today usually make it possible to distinguish harmless lumps that can be left alone or treated medically from cancerous tumors that must be removed.

TESTS FOR THYROID NODULES

There are a number of ways to evaluate a thyroid nodule with laboratory tests and imaging procedures. These are summarized in Table 3 and include the following:

- Blood tests to see if you have an overactive or underactive thyroid

- Imaging studies, which include radioactive-thyroid scans as well as ultrasound pictures, which use sound waves

- Thyroid biopsies, in which a sample of the nodule is removed with a small needle

Many physicians prefer that patients have blood tests and thyroid-imaging studies, and only recommend a biopsy when results indicate that the nodule is a poorly functioning solid lump, which could indicate the presence of cancer rather than a functioning lump or fluid-filled cyst which is rarely cancerous. On the other hand more and more thyroid experts are recommending that their patients have a biopsy as the first test, prior to having any blood tests or thyroid-imaging studies, because imaging studies rarely provide a definite answer about the nature of the nodule. Also, almost all patients who have scans and ultrasound studies end up having a biopsy anyway, since the vast majority of thyroid lumps turn out to be solid and poorly functioning, requiring further evaluation. Therefore, in an era when medical costs have assumed great importance, it is more cost-effective to do a biopsy without first doing thyroid-imaging studies, since a biopsy will be required in most cases. In the rest of this chapter we will describe the evaluation of a patient with a thyroid nodule using the traditional approach of scanning with or without ultrasound, followed by a biopsy, if needed. However, if your physician suggests that a biopsy be done as the first step in your evaluation, it is an equally acceptable approach and is being chosen with greater and greater frequency.

The Traditional Approach

Blood tests that reveal high or low thyroid-hormone levels or the presence of antithyroid antibodies (suggesting the presence of chronic lymphocytic thyroiditis) help to indicate that a lump is probably not cancerous. But a radioiodine thyroid scan may be far more useful, for it provides evidence of the way the nodule itself is functioning.

In order to have a thyroid scan made, you will be given a small amount of radioiodine to swallow in a capsule or in a small amount of water, or else you will receive an injection of a radioactive material called *technetium*. Twenty-four hours later (or twenty minutes later in the case of technetium), a scan picture is made that creates an image of your entire thyroid gland. (Figure 29). The position of your nodule can be located on the scan, making it possible to compare the function of the nodule with that of the surrounding thyroid tissue. In addition the scan provides helpful information about the function of the rest of your thyroid, sometimes showing the presence of abnormal areas elsewhere in the gland (Figure 30). A scan pattern showing the presence of several nodules indicates that you probably have a harmless condition known as multinodular goiter.

In a general way you can think of thyroid nodules as hot (functional) or cold (nonfunctional). A *hot nodule* is one that concentrates radioiodine equal to or more than the sur-

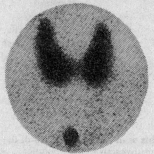

Figure 29 A normal thyroid scan.

rounding thyroid tissue. Occasionally the rest of the thyroid is not even visible on the scan because the hot nodule is making so much thyroid hormone that the function of the rest of the thyroid gland is suppressed (Figure 31). In our experience hot nodules are rarely, if ever, malignant.

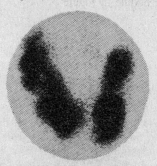

Figure 30 Multinodular goiter.

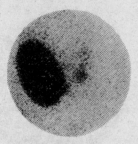

Figure 31 This scan shows almost all of the radioiodine is concentrated in an overactive "hot" nodule.

A *cold nodule* concentrates radioiodine poorly or not at all (Figure 32). Although all cancers are cold, most benign tumors and cysts are also cold. In fact only about 5 to 10 percent of solitary cold nodules prove to be malignant. However, the presence of a cold nodule is always an indication for further evaluation. Moreover, it is more likely to contain cancer if the radioiodine scan shows it to be the only inactive area in an otherwise normal-appearing thyroid gland (like the nodule in Figure 32).

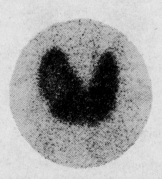

Figure 32 An inactive or "cold" nodule.

FURTHER MANAGEMENT OF THYROID NODULES

Hot nodules can cause hyperthyroidism by producing excessive amounts of thyroid hormones. In general small hot nodules (less than 1 inch in diameter) do not produce hyperthyroidism, but larger ones have a progressively greater chance of producing too much thyroid hormone. Thus your physician can get some idea about the activity of your hot nodule just by measuring its size. If you have a hot nodule, you may not need treatment at all. However, if the nodule is producing even slight elevations in thyroid-hormone levels, therapy may be recommended to protect you from losing calcium from your bones, since it is now recognized that even a slight thyroid-hormone excess can lead to osteoporosis. If no treatment is given, follow-up is important because even a small nodule can, in time, grow and produce too much thyroid hormone. If this occurs, treatment will be recommended to control symptoms of hyperthyroidism (see Chapter 5).

If your nodule is cold on scan, however, your doctor will want to know whether the lump is nonfunctional because it contains cancer, because it is a fluid-filled cyst, or because it is simply one of the harmless types of solid thyroid tumors. Your physician may recommend an ultrasound test, a painless procedure that utilizes sound waves much as radar would to create a picture of the thyroid gland. Cysts appear as dark or "echo-free" areas, quite different from the way solid tumors look. However, a drawback of the ultrasound test is that it cannot determine with certainty whether a solid tumor is harmless or cancerous. The best test to have performed on cold nodules is a fine-needle aspiration biopsy.

THYROID BIOPSY

The term *biopsy* refers to either of two procedures that are performed to get a sample of thyroid tissue for examination under a microscope. To perform the test, your physician will numb the skin of your neck with a local anesthetic and

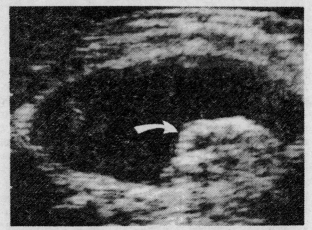

Figure 33 A thyroid cyst as it appears in an ultrasound picture; the dark fluid-filled cyst contains a small amount of thyroid tissue (arrow).

will then insert a needle into your thyroid nodule. In a *fine-needle aspiration* a small number of thyroid cells are withdrawn from the thyroid gland through a small needle attached to a syringe. In contrast, in a *cutting-needle biopsy*, use of a larger hollow needle permits the removal of a core of thyroid tissue for examination. The cutting-needle biopsy is rarely used today because the fine-needle biopsy is very accurate and simpler to perform. These procedures are safe in experienced hands and are normally carried out in a physician's office. A doctor with experience in the fine-needle aspiration technique generally gets very accurate results. However, doctors with little experience may get inconclusive results. Thus if you need a thyroid biopsy, it is likely that your physician will refer you to someone who specializes in the procedure.

About 70 percent of the time, a biopsy will show that a thyroid nodule is benign (harmless). A benign diagnosis usually means that your physician will need only to recheck the nodule in follow-up appointments to be sure that it is not enlarging or causing new symptoms. Sometimes patients are given thyroid hormone medication to take, which may cause the nodule to shrink as discussed later in this chapter. About 5 percent of nodules will show cancer cells in the biopsy specimen. If the nodule contains cancer, your physician will almost certainly recommend that the nodule and some or all of the thyroid be removed in an operation.

About 20 percent of biopsy specimens will be reported as *suspicious*, and about 5 percent are called *nondiagnostic*, because they contain an insufficient amount of tissue for a diagnosis to be made. If your nodule is suspicious, your physician may recommend a period of observation while you take thyroid hormone, to see if the nodule shrinks in size, or immediate surgical removal may be advised. Fortunately the majority of suspicious nodules turn out to be benign. If the biopsy is nondiagnostic, most physicians recommend that the procedure be repeated in order to get an adequate specimen. If this proves to be impossible, a trial of thyroid-hormone therapy or surgical removal will probably be recommended.

It is also possible that particular characteristics of your nodule, or factors such as a history of head or neck irradiation in childhood, may lead your physician to recommend immediate surgical removal of the nodule instead of a biopsy. This step will provide an accurate diagnosis and will of course be a definitive form of treatment as well. But whatever your situation, if you are concerned and want additional information, request a second opinion from another physician about your nodule. In fact your insurance company may require such a consultation if your doctor recommends an operation.

THYROID HORMONE TREATMENT OF THYROID NODULES

If you have several hot and/or cold nodules in your thyroid, you probably have a very common condition known as multinodular goiter (see Chapter 2). These goiters rarely contain cancer. They are made up of hot or cold nodules that produce a characteristic "patchy" uptake of radioiodine

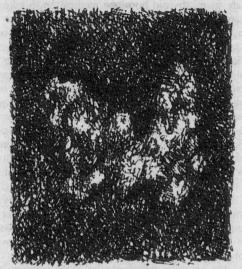

Figure 34 A scan of a multinodular goiter.

throughout the gland in a thyroid-scan picture (Figure 34). If that is your situation, or if you have a single nodule that is too small to biopsy, or one that is located in a part of your thyroid that cannot be biopsied, your physician may choose to observe the nodule for a few months. During the period of observation you may be treated with thyroid-hormone tablets, either to try to shrink the nodule or to shrink the surrounding tissue and thus make the nodule easier to feel. Thyroid hormone pills are often used in this way. They act by "turning off" your pituitary gland's production of thyroid stimulating hormone (TSH). The lack of stimulation by TSH causes some (but not all) benign nodules and all normal thyroid tissue to decrease in size. In fact if your nodule does get smaller during treatment with thyroid hormone pills, that tells your doctor that your nodule is likely to be benign. For this reason many physicians prescribe thyroid hormone to try to shrink nodules that have been found to be benign with a biopsy; if the nodule does get smaller, it is confirmatory evidence that it is harmless.

If you are treated with thyroid hormone, your physician will probably ask you to return periodically for evaluation. One reason for checkups is to be sure that you are not taking an excessive dose. If so, your doctor will probably lower your dose of thyroid and reexamine you at a later date. The TSH blood test is the most accurate way to be sure that your dose of thyroid hormone is correct.

IF THE NODULE PROVES CANCEROUS . . . WHAT THEN?

Even in those rare instances when a cold nodule proves to be a thyroid cancer, it should not necessarily be a cause for alarm. Typically thyroid cancers grow slowly, and most can be completely removed surgically. In those instances when the tumor cannot be entirely removed, it usually responds to treatment with thyroid hormone and radioactive iodine, occasionally supplemented with X-ray treatment and chemotherapy.

There are several types of malignant thyroid tumors. They include *papillary, follicular, Hürthle cell, medullary*, and *anaplastic* cancers. Papillary thyroid cancer is by far the most common, and it is also the variant that tends to occur in individuals who received radiation treatments to the head and neck region in the past. Fortunately this type of thyroid cancer usually is the easiest to cure. It tends to spread only to nearby lymph glands and rarely spreads to other parts of the body. Follicular cancer and Hürthle cell cancer are more likely to spread from the thyroid to distant sites of the body, including the bones, lungs, and liver, so they may be more difficult to control. If you have papillary or follicular thyroid cancer, your physician may order special tests, including chest X-rays, radioiodine scans, and bone scans. Medullary thyroid cancer has several special features, and will be discussed later in this chapter. Anaplastic cancer is the most serious form of thyroid malignancy, and always has a poor outlook. Since treatment of any thyroid cancer can be complicated, your physician may seek advice from a thyroid-cancer specialist or cancer expert.

Recommended treatment will depend on the type and extent of tumor that is present. Generally therapy begins with a thyroid operation that is designed to remove most or all of the thyroid cancer—usually most if not all of the thyroid gland is removed as well. Sometimes surgery is followed by treatment with radioactive iodine to try to eliminate any remaining cancer cells in the thyroid gland. In order to monitor for the recurrence or spread of thyroid cancer, your physician should measure the level of a substance known as *thyroglobulin* in a sample of your blood. Thyroglobulin is a large protein that acts as a storage site for thyroid hormones within the thyroid gland. Normally the amount of thyroglobulin in your blood is small, but it may increase if you have a thyroid cancer that has spread to other body tissues. Thus a high thyroglobulin level in a blood test may mean that the cancer has spread or that cancer once thought cured has recurred. Almost all patients will be placed on lifelong therapy with thyroid-hormone tablets. Just as in the case of benign nodules and normal thyroid tissue, many forms of thyroid cancer are dependent on TSH for growth. Hence thyroid hormone is administered in an effort to suppress the secretion of TSH from the pituitary and thereby prevent growth of the thyroid cancer. With most thyroid cancer a complete cure is common, and the outlook with treatment is excellent.

A SPECIAL KIND OF THYROID CANCER

About 10 percent of thyroid cancers are somewhat unusual tumors known as medullary carcinomas. These tumors may be discovered as a single hard lump in the neck like other forms of thyroid cancer. In such cases they should be evaluated like other thyroid nodules, and often they can be successfully treated by surgical removal. In some patients, however, these tumors develop as part of an inherited disorder, and in such individuals more than one medullary cancer can usually be found within the thyroid gland. Patients with this condition may also develop tumors of the adrenal glands (which can cause high blood pressure) and parathyroid glands (which can raise the blood-calcium level). In some patients nerve tumors *(neuromas)* may also appear.

Medullary thyroid cancer cells produce a hormone known as *calcitonin*, which can be detected by a blood test. Calcitonin measurements are helpful in several ways. First, the presence of calcitonin in the blood tells us that the patient has a medullary cancer. Second, if it is still present in the patient's blood after thyroid surgery has been completed, it means that not all of the tumor has been removed and that more tumor treatment is needed. Finally, if a patient has the inherited type of medullary thyroid cancer, physicians can use calcitonin blood tests to find out which relatives have the same condition before the tumor has fully developed. This is vitally important, for those relatives who have the best opportunity of being cured of this cancer are those in whom evidence of the tumor is found in childhood, before spread of the tumor cells from the thyroid has occurred.

Obviously medullary thyroid carcinoma is a tumor with many characteristics that make it different from other types of cancer. Therefore, if you or a member of your family has this type of thyroid problem, it is very important that you find out from your physician whether other family members should also be tested for evidence of this disorder.

TABLE 2

Characteristics of Cancerous and Benign Thyroid Nodules (History and Physical Examination)

The likelihood that a nodule is a cancer is increased if:	*The likelihood that a nodule is benign is increased if:*
HISTORY	
the patient is a child or adolescent.	the patient is an adult.
the patient is male.	the patient is female.
the patient has had x-ray treatment to the head, neck, or chest in childhood.	the patient has symptoms of an overactive or underactive thyroid.
the patient has noticed rapid enlargement of the nodule.	the patient has a strong family history of benign thyroid diseases such as chronic lymphocytic thyroiditis or multinodular goiter.
the patient has noticed a change in voice, hoarseness, or trouble in swallowing, suggesting compression of nearby neck structures.	
PHYSICAL EXAMINATION	
a single lump is felt in the thyroid.	more than one lump is felt in the thyroid.
the lump is "fixed" (attached) to the tissues around it.	no lymph node enlargement can be found.
the nearby neck lymph glands are enlarged.	the rest of the thyroid feels abnormal (firm, enlarged, irregular, etc).
the rest of the thyroid feels normal.	

TABLE 3

Characteristics of Cancerous and Benign Thyroid Nodules (Thyroid Tests)

	The likelihood that a nodule is a cancer is increased if:	The likelihood that a nodule is benign is increased if:
Thyroid hormone blood level	is normal.	is high or low (but often will be normal).
Antithyroid antibody in blood	is absent.	is present.
Radioiodine scan	shows that lump is "cold" or "cool" concentrating radioiodine poorly.	shows that lump concentrates radioiodine.
Thyroid ultrasound	shows solid tumor.	shows a cyst (but often benign tumors will be solid).
Thyroid needle biopsy	reveals cancer cells.	reveals cyst fluid or benign thyroid cells.

A THYROID BIOPSY

by S.S.

The doctor's quiet and calm manner set the tone for the procedure. First he examined my neck with his fingers. This didn't hurt at all. Then he drew a picture on paper showing me where my thyroid lump was in my thyroid gland. He explained what he was going to do and why it was important to do it. We then walked into his examining room. I unbuttoned the top three or four buttons on my shirt, and lay on my back on his examining table. The nurse put pillows under my shoulders so that my head hung back. It felt like I was upside down. This position exposed my neck area, which was washed with alcohol. The doctor told me he was going to inject Novocain into my neck. The needle felt like a pinprick or a mosquito bite.

After a few minutes the Novocain had numbed my neck, and the doctor proceeded with the biopsy itself. This meant that he put a needle through the numb skin on my neck into my thyroid lump. The only feeling on my neck during the procedure was slight pressure. There was absolutely no pain or discomfort. Toward the end I felt a little dizzy and clammy, probably due to my nervousness and to the fact that my head was extended backward over a pillow. The doctor kept explaining and talking to me during the whole procedure so that I always knew what was going on and never felt afraid.

After the biopsy was over, I held a gauze pad against the place on my neck where the biopsy had been done. The pillow under my shoulders was removed, and I was asked to lie quietly for about ten minutes. During this time all my dizziness went away. Soon the nurse put a small bandage on the biopsy place on my neck. Then I got up and walked into the doctor's outer office, where I waited for a few more minutes. Then I left his office, drove home, and ate supper. There was no pain, discomfort, or dizziness.

Later that night I noticed a sore feeling as if I had a slight bruise on my neck. There was also slight swelling where the biopsy had been done. However, there was no real pain or serious discomfort.

A THYROID NODULE DISCOVERED, TESTED, AND REMOVED

by H. J.

During a physical examination, my doctor told me he thought he felt a lump, or "nodule," in my thyroid gland. Because of this he took a blood sample to measure my thyroid-hormone level and ordered a thyroid scan. My blood test was normal, but the scan, which was made using a small dose of radioactive iodine that I had swallowed the day before, showed that there was a nodule as suspected and that it was not "functioning." That means it did not take up iodine as the rest of the thyroid gland did, appearing instead like an empty hole in the scan picture [see Figure 35].

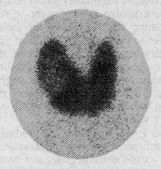

Figure 35 An inactive or "cold" nodule.

The next step was a thyroid biopsy. This was performed by a surgeon and was done to learn what kind of thyroid tissue was in the nodule, and thus determine whether it had to be removed in an operation.

I was relieved to discover that a biopsy was not much more difficult or painful for me than having a blood sample taken. The surgeon asked me to loosen a few buttons of my shirt and lie on my back with my neck extended over a bunched-up pillow to better expose the front of my neck where the thyroid is located. After cleaning my neck with alcohol he numbed the skin with a local anesthetic. After the skin was numb, he inserted a needle into the thyroid nodule, and through the needle he was able to obtain the biopsy specimen. During the biopsy I felt a pressure sensation in my neck but no pain. I also had an urge to cough (but suppressed it) when the surgeon pressed on my windpipe. Afterward I held a cotton bandage on the biopsy site for about five minutes. Then my "wound" was covered with a small bandage. I got up without any ill effects and went home to await the report of the biopsy.

After examining the biopsy specimen, my physicians agreed that an operation was indicated. The surgeon told me about the operation that he planned to do—a "partial thyroidectomy." This meant that only the left lobe of the thyroid, which contained the nodule, was to be removed. I was told that more extensive surgery might be required if the examination during surgery revealed the presence of more widespread disease than expected. I learned that I would be admitted the day before surgery for a physical examination and tests of my general health. I was told that I could expect a sore throat for several days after surgery, but that I would be able to eat breakfast the morning after surgery. I was to plan to take two to three weeks off work after surgery because I would feel tired.

A week later I was admitted to the hospital. In the afternoon, routine preoperative tests were performed, including a chest X ray, an electrocardiogram, and blood and urine tests. That evening an anesthesiologist came to my room and told me a little about what would happen. He said that I could not eat or drink after midnight. If I wanted, I could get an injection to relax me on the morning of surgery before being taken to the operating room. He told me that an IV would be put in my arm through which I would be given an injection to put me to sleep. After I was asleep, a plastic tube would be inserted through my mouth into my windpipe in order to give me oxygen and anesthetic gases during the operation. He said that I would feel groggy for a few hours after I woke up and that I might be nauseated.

Things went pretty much as everyone had said. I slept remarkably well the night before surgery, although I was a little anxious. I was wide awake and hungry the morning of surgery (although of course I couldn't have anything to eat). A surgical orderly dressed in a scrub suit, hair net, and mask came into my room with a stretcher for me to lie on. He took me through various corridors to the operating-room area and then parked my stretcher in a little cubicle outside the room in which my operation would take place. Soon an operating-room nurse and a nurse-anesthetist came to my side. They asked me my name and whether I had any allergies, as well as a few of the other questions I had been asked before, just to make sure everything was in order. Finally, the nurse-anesthetist started the IV in my arm. Shortly thereafter I spotted my surgeon standing nearby. After speaking briefly with my surgeon and hearing some encouraging words from the people around me, I was given an intravenous injection of morphine that made my whole body tingle and began to make me drowsy. At this point I was wheeled into the operating room itself. I was still awake and set about arranging myself on the operating table, but the masked faces of the people around me gradually drifted out of sight as sodium pentothal was injected into my IV and I fell asleep.

When I awoke, I was lying on a bed in the recovery room. Here I was to spend the next few hours to be sure that there were no complications from the operation following surgery. I had a very sore throat and it was hard for me to swallow. I felt very drugged. I could open my eyes for about five seconds, recognize people, read the clock on the wall, even talk, but then I would drift back to sleep. I did not need any pain medication during this time. After about four hours I was taken back to my hospital room, where I drifted in and out of sleep until about nine P.M. Then, about eight hours after surgery and still with a sore throat and difficulty in swallowing, I woke up for several hours, although I felt very weak. I was able to walk to the bathroom with assistance, although it took several attempts before I was able to empty my obviously full bladder—an effect of the anesthetic drugs. I was able to sip ginger ale through a straw, although every swallow hurt. I slept on and off throughout the night, and I refused pain medication because the grogginess and nausea from the drugs seemed worse than the sore throat from surgery.

I was considerably more awake the next morning and managed to swallow a soft breakfast. My IV came out (thank goodness—my hand was hurting). Then a small rubber drain in my neck was removed, and a suture was tied where it had been (all painless). During the rest of my hospital stay my throat gradually became less and less sore. On the second day my stitches were removed and I went home. I felt weak, and tired easily for about a week, but had recovered full strength by two weeks after surgery. The swelling around the site of surgery and the mild tenderness over the left side of my neck (where the nodule and thyroid lobe were removed) also resolved during that time.

SUMMARY

In summary, physicians have at their disposal ways to accurately determine the cause of a thyroid nodule. In most instances tests will show that the nodule is harmless and surgery unnecessary. When studies suggest that cancer is likely to be present in a thyroid nodule, surgery alone may be curative, though other forms of treatment are available when needed.

CHAPTER ELEVEN

The Thyroid and Radiation

It must be appreciated that the usual course of growth of a thyroid cancer in young people is slow, and that the risk of death from thyroid cancer is extremely low. This risk must be balanced against the unavoidable risks which are associated with any medical intervention, including the development of undue anxiety, the cost and inconveniences of examinations, further radiation exposure, and the risk of surgery. Any medical procedures must be done after full and careful evaluation, recognizing that hasty action is very rarely required.

—From DeGroot LJ, Frohman LA, Kaplan EL, Refeto HS,
*Summary and conclusions of the conference on radiation-associated
thyroid cancer,* University of Chicago, 1976

In the 1920s physicians began to use radiation (X rays) to treat noncancerous disorders. One of the more common problems that was treated in this manner was an enlargement of the *thymus* gland in newborns. The thymus gland is located behind the breastbone and is important for normal immune function. Other conditions treated in this manner included enlarged tonsils or adenoids, birthmarks, whooping cough, acne, and ringworm of the scalp. Treatment was given by means of an X-ray machine ("external beam irradiation") or by placing radioactive material, such as radium, directly in or on the tissue to be treated.

For many years radiation was considered good medical therapy for some of these problems. For example deafness was improved when radium treatments shrank enlarged lymph tissue compressing the internal ear canal. Acne could be markedly improved by radiation, resulting in less facial scarring. In short, radiation therapy was used because it seemed safe and effective. Unfortunately the thyroid gland, located as it is at the front of the neck, often received radiation inadvertently during treatment for these conditions.

In the 1950s physicians began to notice an increased number of benign and malignant thyroid tumors among patients who had been given radiation therapy years earlier. The fact that the radiation had caused the thyroid tumors was substantiated when it was found that many individuals exposed to atomic-bomb radiation or fallout also developed thyroid tumors in later years. When these facts became known, these forms of radiation therapy were of course discontinued. Nevertheless it is estimated that between one and two million people across the United States received radiation treatments in childhood or adolescence between 1920 and the early 1960s. Subsequent large-scale studies of thyroid-cancer frequency in radiated and nonradiated control groups have established beyond doubt the relationship between radiation exposure and thyroid cancer.

If you or a member of your family received such X-ray treatments in the past, it is possible that the hospital at which you were treated has tried to contact you to inform you about your radiation exposure. Unfortunately since people tend to move many times during their lifetimes, and since women may change their names as well as their addresses, hospitals have been unable to reach many of these patients. Therefore if you have not been contacted but think you have received X-ray treatment, please try to contact the hospital where your treatment was given. If the medical record of that treatment is still available, it will be forwarded to you promptly upon your request and will be helpful to the physician you go to for your follow-up examination. Here is an example of an appropriate letter to a hospital:

Medical Records Department
Your Local Hospital
Any Street
Your Town, State, Zip

To the Medical Records Librarian:

I believe that I received X-ray treatment for an enlarged thymus gland a few days after I was born. Please send me my medical information about treatment given, including the dose of X ray received, the number of treatments given, and the part of my body that was radiated.

My personal information is as follows:
Name at the time of treatment: Rebecca C. Smith
Date of birth: March 21, 1926
Exact date of treatment: Unknown, probably late March 1926
Address at that time: 27 Charles Street, Boston, Massachusetts
Mother's name: Mary Louise Smith
Father's name: Francis Clark Smith
Obstetrician: Grover Thornton, M.D.
Pediatrician: George Jones, M.D.

Very sincerely yours,

Rebecca Smith Jacobsen
Your Street
Your Town, State, Zip

It would be a good idea to enclose a stamped, self-addressed envelope, though under normal circumstances this would be provided by the hospital. In most cases there will be no charge for this service.

Should you be unable to find the appropriate information in this manner, or if the treatment was performed in a doctor's office, we would recommend that you make an effort to contact one of the physicians who treated you. Give the physician your name and address as it was at the time, since the information will be needed to locate your medical record. You may find that the doctor who treated you has died or moved away, or that your records have been lost or destroyed: but try to find them, for they can provide helpful information for the physician who will examine you.

If you had radiation treatments given to your head, neck, or chest, you may have many questions about their effect on you and what you should do about it. The following section should help to answer some of the most commonly asked questions.

HOW COMMON IS THE APPEARANCE OF THYROID CANCER FOLLOWING EARLIER IRRADIATION?

If you had radiation treatment for an enlarged thymus, acne, or some other condition near your thyroid gland, you are more likely to develop thyroid cancer someday than someone who has no history of radiation treatment. Medical surveys suggest that your overall thyroid-cancer risk is somewhere between 2 and 12 percent, compared with an annual incidence of 0.004 percent in the general population. Although your risk increases with increased amounts of radiation, we have not observed an increased risk of thyroid cancer in patients who had hyperthyroidism treated by radioactive iodine. Here the thyroid receives far greater amounts of radiation from the radioactive iodine treatment (from 4000 to 12,000 rads), and yet thirty to forty years' follow-up of such patients has failed to demonstrate that they have an increased risk for thyroid cancer. However, recent reports have shown that high doses of external radiation to the head and neck area, such as that given for certain forms of cancer, may cause thyroid tumors as well as hypothyroidism at a later time. There is also good evidence that radiation to the thyroid from thyroid scans using radioactive iodine is not associated with thyroid cancer. We do not know why cancer is associated with low doses of X rays administered externally but not with low doses of radiation from radioactive iodine taken internally.

WHAT OTHER FACTORS BESIDES THE AMOUNT OF RADIATION YOU RECEIVED INCREASE YOUR CHANCES OF DEVELOPING THYROID CANCER?

Clearly one important factor is the part of your body that was treated by X rays. Some patients received radiation by means of small pieces of radium placed directly in or on tissues to be treated. Radiation of tonsils or adenoid tissue was sometimes carried out in this manner. If that is your situation, your thyroid gland probably got less radiation effect than the thyroid of someone whose X-ray treatment was given directly to the front of the neck, where the thyroid is located. In fact one study has suggested that people subjected to radium implants as children develop thyroid cancer at a frequency no greater than the general population.

Gender is another factor that is associated with the risk of developing thyroid cancer in irradiated populations. We do not know why, but girls and women develop thyroid cancer at a higher rate than boys and men. However, this also occurs when there is no history of irradiation, so it is perhaps logical that the same tendency would be noted in people exposed to radiation.

Age also appears to play a role in this process. The younger a person was at the time of radiation exposure, the more likely it is that a cancer will develop, probably because the growing thyroid gland of a child is more susceptible to the damaging effects of radiation than the thyroid of an adult.

Another factor currently under investigation involves hypothyroidism. If a patient had radiation and subsequently developed hypothyroidism (thyroid failure) as a second disorder, it is possible that the hypothyroidism itself may increase the risk of later development of thyroid nodules and thyroid cancer. This is because the pituitary gland secretes thyroid-simulating hormone in response to the hypothyroidism. TSH is thought to be one factor that can cause thyroid tumors to develop. Experiments with animals suggest that is the case, although it has never been proved in human beings. Nevertheless because of our experience with irradiated animals, if even a slight decrease in thyroid function occurs in someone with a history of childhood irradiation, it is very important to raise his or her thyroid blood level to normal through the administration of thyroid-hormone tablets.

It is clear that the risk of developing thyroid problems stays with a person for his or her entire lifetime. Thyroid cancer has been detected in exposed individuals as long as fifty years after the X-ray treatments were administered.

However, it has been about thirty years since physicians stopped using this form of treatment, so it is likely that cancers due to radiation will decrease in the years to come.

HAVE OTHER KINDS OF MEDICAL PROBLEMS APPEARED IN IRRADIATED PATIENTS?

Other kinds of neck tumors have been found in patients who received childhood irradiation. These include tumors of the parotid (mumps) glands, which are located below the ears, as well as other salivary glands located beneath the jaw. In addition tumors of the parathyroid glands, located behind the thyroid, develop more commonly in irradiated patients than in the general population, as are other rare tumors of the neck region. We are continuing to look for other associated medical problems, but as yet no other medical relationships have been firmly established.

Hypothyroidism and thyroid nodules are common occurrences in patients receiving large doses of external radiation for tumors of the neck and chest region, such as in Hodgkin's disease. It is therefore very important that patients who receive radiotherapy to this area have their thyroid function checked periodically for the rest of their lives. In fact many experts recommend that these patients be started on thyroid-hormone supplementation as a preventative measure, since the risk of developing hypothyroidism and/or thyroid tumors is so high.

Paradoxically a number of studies have shown that patients who get X-ray treatment to the head and neck area are at greater risk for the development of *hyperthyroidism* due to Graves' disease.* The cause of this is unclear, but it may be that damage or injury to the thyroid leads to an abnormality of the body's immune system, in which the thyroid becomes a target for antibodies capable of stimulating it to become overactive (see Chapter 4).

*Hancock SL, Cox RS, McDougall IR. Thyroid Diseases After Treatment of Hodgkin's Disease. *New England Journal of Medicine* 1991; 325: 599–605.

WHAT SORT OF MEDICAL EXAMINATION IS ADVISED FOR PATIENTS WHO HAVE HAD CHILDHOOD IRRADIATION?

If you have had childhood irradiation, you should be seen by your physician for yearly checkups. Your physician will examine your neck to determine whether thyroid nodules are present and also to look for any abnormalities of your parotid glands, salivary glands, or lymph nodes that might suggest the presence of a tumor.

If a thyroid abnormality is found, a thyroid scan should be performed, both to evaluate the function of suspicious lumps and also to look for areas of diminished thyroid activity within your gland that could not be felt by your physician. A thyroid scan, using techniques currently available, adds very little radiation to your already radiated thyroid gland. As explained in Chapter 1 the thyroid receives a dose of 1.1 to 4.4 rads from radioiodine (^{123}I) and 1 to 2 rads from radioactive technetium (^{99m}Tc). Your physician may not perform such a scan on you, however, if your thyroid feels normal and you are willing to return for periodic examinations.

Your physician will probably perform a blood test to measure your level of thyroid hormone (T4) as well as your level of pituitary thyroid-stimulating hormone (TSH) to look for evidence of hypothyroidism. Your physician might also measure the level of thyroglobulin in your blood. Thyroglobulin is a protein made by your thyroid gland; recent studies have shown that even when no abnormality of the thyroid can be palpated by a physician, patients with an elevation of thyroglobulin have a greater risk of developing thyroid nodules in the future.

IF YOUR MEDICAL EXAMINATION REVEALS THE PRESENCE OF A THYROID NODULE . . . WHAT NEXT?

If your doctor feels a thyroid nodule and it shows diminished function on a thyroid scan (Figure 36), it should be either biopsied or entirely removed to be sure that it is not cancerous. Fortunately thyroid cancers that develop as a result of irradiation do not appear to be any more aggressive than thyroid cancer that occurs without irradiation; in fact thyroid cancer, whether related to radiation or not, is usually one of the most curable kinds of cancer. In contrast, nodules that appear to function normally or show an increased uptake of radioactive iodine on scan do not necessarily need to be removed, although they should be followed carefully and reexamined in one year (or sooner, at the discretion of the physician).

Further treatment depends on the results of the T4 and TSH blood tests. If these show that hypothyroidism is present, treatment will be with thyroid hormone tablets in in-

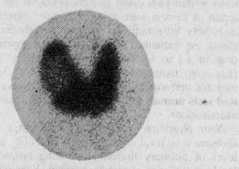

Figure 36   An inactive or "cold" nodule.

creasing doses until the serum TSH becomes low (see Chapter 6). If hyperthyroidism is diagnosed, your doctor will discuss various treatments with you. Your doctor may order a test to measure the level of *thyroglobulin* in your blood. If the thyroglobulin level is elevated, your doctor might order an ultrasound examination, which is a sensitive test that can detect extremely small thyroid nodules; he or she may also decide to see you more frequently for routine follow-up visits to be sure that you do not develop a thyroid tumor.

WHAT SORT OF CONTINUED HEALTH CHECKUPS SHOULD YOU HAVE IF YOU WERE TREATED WITH RADIATION IN CHILDHOOD?

The nature of your follow-up evaluation depends on what was found at the time of your initial evaluation. If no nodules are found on your initial examination and your thyroid blood tests and scan are normal, you can simply have yearly checkups by your family physician, with thyroid blood tests to be sure that you do not develop hypothyroidism. It is not recommended that a thyroid scan be done every year.

On the other hand, if your initial thyroid evaluation revealed the presence of one or more small nodules that are too small to biopsy, a different follow-up is usually indicated. If there is no evidence that the nodule is functioning excessively your physician will probably attempt to suppress its growth with thyroid hormone tablets. As explained in Chapter 10, this treatment raises your blood level of thyroid hormone, which blocks the release of thyroid-stimulating hormone from your pituitary. TSH tends to make many thyroid nodules grow larger, and shutting off TSH sometimes makes thyroid nodules shrink. If there is no diminution in size after three to six months of treatment, however, your physician may recommend that the nodule be biopsied or removed surgically.

It should be stressed that your risk of developing thyroid tumors following childhood irradiation does not disappear with time. Therefore you must continue to have yearly checkups of your thyroid gland throughout your lifetime.

CONTROVERSIAL "CANCERS"

In our discussion about thyroid tumors and cancers, we have been referring in general to nodules that are large enough to be felt on physical examination. One of the most hotly contested issues in the field of thyroid cancer has to do with the presence in many thyroid glands of very small tumors that are less than 1 centimeter (¼ inch) in size, many so small that they can be detected only with a microscope. And though many of these abnormal areas look like cancers, there is no proof that they actually ever develop into a growing, spreading cancer. Since they can occur in individuals who have never had childhood irradiation, as well as in those who were exposed to X ray treatments in childhood, we see no reason to recommend removal of the thyroid gland simply because of the possible presence of such areas and a history of childhood irradiation.

Unfortunately there is no evidence that taking thyroid hormone to suppress TSH secretion by the pituitary gland prevents the development of thyroid cancer in adults who were irradiated as children many decades earlier. Following radiation to the neck region for cancers such as Hodgkin's disease, discussed above, thyroid hormone is begun soon after the radiation treatment, but in a case of childhood irradiation for benign disease, when thyroid medication is started decades after the radiation exposure, it simply does not appear to be effective.

But if you had childhood irradiation for benign disease, starting thyroid medication now is not likely to prevent your developing thyroid cancer. On the other hand, it may inhibit growth of benign nodules and thus simplify your follow-up examination.

WHAT ABOUT NUCLEAR-REACTOR ACCIDENTS, ATOMIC-WEAPONS TESTING, AND THE THYROID?

As a by-product of the process of producing atomic energy, all nuclear reactors produce various forms of radioactive iodine, called *isotopes*. Due to spontaneous loss of radioactivity, known as *decay*, some isotopes of iodine last only a few seconds or a few hours, while others last for longer periods of time. One isotope, called ^{129}I, lasts for 100 million years! Fortunately its radioactivity is so weak that it is barely measurable. In terms of thyroid disease the most important radioiodine isotope is ^{131}I, which decays to half its strength in about eight days.

In a nuclear reactor accident various isotopes of radioiodine are released in the form of a radioactive cloud. The radiation is then blown downwind, where it settles on grass and other vegetation and is then eaten by cows and other livestock. It ultimately appears in their milk. Infants and children ingest the contaminated milk, and the radioiodine is eventually concentrated by their thyroid glands. Unfortunately the thyroids of children may be more sensitive to radiation than those of adults. First, the thyroid cells of a child are growing rapidly, which makes them more susceptible to radiation damage. Second, a child's thyroid has a smaller volume than that of an adult, so each cell receives a larger dose of radiation from any given amount of radioiodine.

The world's most infamous nuclear accident occurred in April 1986 at a reactor in Chernobyl, in the former Soviet Union. At that time approximately 40 million *Curies* of radioiodine were released into the atmosphere. (A Curie is a measure of radioactivity. A typical dose of ^{131}I used to treat hyperthyroidism is 10 millicuries, or $\frac{1}{100}$th of a Curie.) In comparison a previous accident at the Windscale reactor in Great Britain in 1957 released about 20,000 Curies, and the much-publicized incident at Pennsylvania's Three Mile Island facility in 1979 released less than 20 Curies.

Not all radiation exposure comes from nuclear reactor accidents. Inhabitants of the Marshall Islands in the South Pacific were exposed inadvertently to radioactive fallout from an atomic test at Bikini Atoll in 1954, and residents of southwestern Utah living downwind from the Nevada Test Site were exposed to radioiodine from 1951 through 1962. More recently it became known that residents living near a nuclear-weapons facility in Hanford, Washington, were exposed to radioiodine from 1944 through the early 1970s, with the largest exposures occurring between 1944 and 1947.

From long-term follow-up studies of the Marshall Islanders, we know that people, especially children, exposed to radioactive iodine from atomic testing can develop thyroid tumors. There is also evidence that people living in Utah have developed thyroid nodules. And there are recent reports from the Ukraine and Beylorus that thyroid cancer is now being diagnosed with greater frequency in children who lived in the Chernobyl area, but these observations have yet to be confirmed.

For technical reasons involving the design of the reactor core, the release of enormous quantities of radioactive iodine on the scale of Chernobyl or Windscale, is virtually impossible at the nuclear power plants found in this country. Nevertheless citizens who live near nuclear facilities are appropriately concerned about the possible consequences of a release of radioiodine into the air. The following guidelines, suggested by the American Thyroid Association, should be followed in the unlikely event of a nuclear accident in which radioiodine is released: People should not drink fresh liquids (for example, juices, milk, or water) or eat fresh foods. Canned and bottled liquids and previously prepared foods are safe, as is water from underground springs or well water.

A drug known as *potassium iodide* has been shown to block the concentration of harmful radioactive iodine in the thyroid. Although some public health officials have advocated that populations exposed to radioactive iodine take potassium iodide for protection, this practice is controversial, since potassium iodide itself can have adverse health effects in a small number of people. Potassium iodide would have to be taken for several weeks—while it would protect the thyroid, some susceptible people might develop hypothyroidism as a result of taking the drug for this extended period of time. Therefore the issue has not been settled, and it continues to be discussed by governmental agencies, especially the Nuclear Regulatory Commission and the Federal Emergency Management Administration.*

Work is continuing at medical centers all over the world to understand all of the controversial areas mentioned within this chapter. Every effort is being made by groups like the American Thyroid Association, the Endocrine Society, the Thyroid Foundation of America, and the American Cancer Society to keep you and your physician well informed as the state of our knowledge improves.

---

*D. Becker, "Reactor Accidents: Public Health Strategies and Their Medical Implications," *Journal of the American Medical Association* 258 (1987): 649–654.

SUMMARY

In summary, radioactive iodine used to test the thyroid does not pose a health risk. Similarly, the low doses of radioactive iodine used to treat Graves' disease have not been shown to cause thyroid cancer or other problems.

On the other hand, external radiation and larger amounts of radioactive iodine which may be released in nuclear reactor accidents may pose serious health risks. Fortunately, organizations like the Nuclear Regulatory Commission, and many groups of health professionals who specialize in caring for individuals with thyroid problems, are constantly reviewing and updating guidelines for the follow-up of patients with these higher radiation exposures.

CHAPTER TWELVE

Thyroid Trouble in Children

If your child's thyroid is not working properly, it is likely to have different effects than it would if an adult had the same problem. This is because your child is growing and developing, and growth and development can be changed by a thyroid that is either overactive (hyperthyroid) or underactive (hypothyroid).

In addition, thyroid trouble can be more difficult to recognize in a child than in an adult. Children are less likely to complain of feeling sick or to ask for help. They do not know what "normal" is, so even older children may simply accept the emotional and physical symptoms of a thyroid problem as "normal" for them. Therefore it's usually up to someone else to recognize thyroid diseases when they occur in children. Indeed, an increase in irritability or hyperactivity noticed by a parent, friend, or teacher, or a change in growth rate noted by a parent or pediatrician may be the clue that leads to the discovery of a thyroid problem in a child.

Finally, since some thyroid disorders are inherited, we would like to stress one very important point: If someone in the family has thyroid trouble now or has had a thyroid problem in the past, be sure to tell your child's physician about it. If it is the type of thyroid trouble that can be inherited, you will have alerted the physician to be watchful for that problem in your child.

GOITER IN CHILDHOOD

Anytime the thyroid grows larger than normal, it is called a *goiter*. A goiter may appear at any age but is especially common in girls about the time their menstrual cycles begin.

If your child develops a goiter, it is possible that he or she is still healthy and no important thyroid problem exists. On the other hand, most goiters that appear in children over six years of age are caused by low-grade inflammation of the thyroid gland known as *chronic lymphocytic thyroiditis*, or *Hashimoto's disease*. In adults this condition is a common cause of thyroid failure (see Chapter 7). Occasionally a goiter may be the first sign of some other thyroid problem. For example your child's thyroid may be overactive, or it may be enlarged due to inflammation associated with a viral infection.

Therefore if you notice a goiter in your child, you should take him or her to a physician for a checkup. By examining the child and obtaining a blood test, the doctor can tell if the thyroid gland is overactive or underactive. Either of these thyroid conditions may interfere with a child's growth and development, but treating them will correct the thyroid-hormone level and restore the growth pattern to normal.

Even if the results of the examination and the thyroid tests in a child with a goiter are normal, that does not mean necessarily that the goiter can be forgotten. Rather, the physician will probably reexamine and retest your child at a later time to be sure a change in thyroid function has not occurred.

Rarely, a child's neck will have a swelling that appears to be a generalized enlargement of the entire thyroid gland, but may actually be caused by an enlarged overlying fat pad or by growth of one or more lumps or nodules in the thyroid. The enlarged fat pad, which can be recognized by the fact that it does not move up and down with the Adam's apple when the child swallows, is of no significance. In the case of nodules, however, medical evaluation as outlined later in this chapter is very important and should be carried out promptly. Although most nodules prove to be harmless cysts or benign tumors, occasionally they contain thyroid cancer or reflect a change of thyroid function. Such conditions can and should be treated.

THE OVERACTIVE THYROID IN CHILDHOOD

One of the best-understood forms of thyroid trouble in children is the increased thyroid activity that affects some newborn babies and is known as *neonatal hyperthyroidism*. This condition is rare, occurring only in infants born of mothers with hyperthyroidism caused by Graves' disease. It is due to the passage of chemical substances called *stimulating antibodies* from the mother's blood across the placenta to her unborn baby. When these substances get into the baby's blood stream, they may cause the baby's thyroid to make too much thyroid hormone.

Fortunately this type of hyperthyroidism in a newborn baby lasts only as long as the mother's thyroid antibodies remain in the baby's blood stream, usually from three to twelve weeks. Moreover, the condition is usually mild, since most women who have an overactive thyroid do not have very high blood levels of the thyroid stimulators. Occasionally a mother will have such high levels of the stimulators that her baby will be born with prominent eyes, irritability, flushing of the skin, and a fast pulse—all characteristics of an overactive thyroid at any age. In addition these babies may have tremendous appetites but not gain weight. A goiter is common but may not be obvious at birth.

In its mildest form this disease may require no treatment and will subside by itself in time. However, if the baby is seriously ill, treatment with iodine and an antithyroid drug such as propylthiouracil may be required to control the overactive thyroid gland. If more rapid control of symptoms is required, treatment with a *beta-adrenergic blocking drug*, such as atenolol or propranolol may be helpful. The drug works by blocking the action of the high thyroid hormone levels on the baby's body. Thyroid surgery is rarely if ever needed, even if the baby has a very large thyroid, for treatment with iodine usually causes the gland to shrink rapidly in size. This is fortunate, since a thyroid operation would be extremely difficult in so tiny a patient. Treatment can usually be discontinued in a few weeks, since the mother's thyroid antibodies soon disappear from the baby's blood stream.

Even though this condition is extremely rare, a pregnant woman who has hyperthyroidism or who has been hyperthyroid in the past should alert the obstetrician about her thyroid problem *during the pregnancy* so that her doctor will be prepared to look for a thyroid abnormality in the baby.

Hyperthyroidism that occurs in children after the newborn period is very much like hyperthyroidism in adults. However, children generally do not complain of such things as having too much energy or feeling nervous, so it may be hard to tell if your child is sick with an overactive thyroid, even though you may be exhausted by a hyperactive and restless child who never seems to need a nap (Figure 37). Quite often the *only* clue that a problem exists will be a sudden growth spurt that makes a child with an overactive thyroid suddenly grow taller. A pediatrician who keeps careful records of the child's body measurements may no-

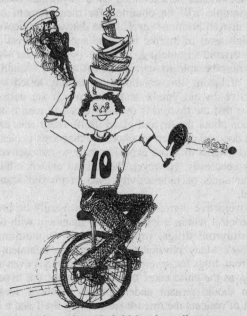

Figure 37 A hyperthyroid child has boundless energy.

tice such a change, but more often parents become aware of a sudden increase in growth when their child rapidly outgrows new clothes.

There are other clues by which we can recognize hyperthyroidism. Virtually all hyperthyroid children have a goiter and prominent eyes. Other common signs of thyroid overactivity include a rapid pulse, nervousness, increased sweating, and a dislike for hot weather. Parents may notice a deterioration of school performance, and the teacher may report that the child doesn't pay attention in class. Rapid growth of fingernails may lead to accumulation of dirt under irregular nail margins. Shaky hands may cause clumsiness and poor handwriting, while weak shoulder and thigh muscles may be apparent in play or sports. Emotional disturbances may be seen, and parents commonly note that even a gentle reprimand brings forth a flood of tears.

If you suspect that your child has an overactive thyroid, he or she should be examined by a physician. Usually a blood sample will be obtained for measurement of the child's thyroid hormone level. If the diagnosis is confirmed by a high level of thyroid hormone and a low level of pituitary thyroid-stimulating hormone (see Chapter 4), the doctor may be able to start treatment at once. Adults suspected of having this condition are usually tested with a radioactive-thyroid uptake and scan, which are performed to prove that the thyroid is overactive and to gain more information about the thyroid gland itself. These tests are not always done on children in whom the diagnosis is clear; the physician wants to avoid exposing them to radioactive substances needlessly. However, there is no evidence that the small amounts of radioactivity used in thyroid scans are harmful.

An overactive thyroid in a child can usually be brought under control within a few weeks by treatment with one of the antithyroid drugs: propylthiouracil or methimazole (Tapazole). Many physicians will continue treatment with antithyroid drugs for several months, sometimes even years. As long as the child takes the drugs reliably, the hyperthyroidism should remain under control. In about 30 to 50 percent of patients the disease subsides by itself and a *spontaneous remission* occurs.

If this is the form of treatment chosen for your child, you should know something about the possible side effects from the drugs. Some children will develop an allergic reaction to the medications, usually manifested as fever, itching, hives, or a red skin rash. Very rarely these antithyroid drugs may produce a more serious problem, such as jaundice or a lowering or even the complete disappearance of certain of the child's white blood cells *(neutrophils)*, which help to protect the child from infections. Therefore if your child is taking one of these drugs and develops fever, itching, hives, a skin rash, or evidence of an infection (such as sore throat, sore mouth, or fever), the child should stop taking the drug and the physician should be notified at once. If the doctor finds that your child is allergic to the antithyroid drug, another form of treatment will be recommended. On the other hand, if the problem is a fever from an infection, the child may be able to continue drug treatment even while the infection is being treated, provided the neutrophil count is normal.

Fortunately antithyroid drugs do not usually cause serious problems, and most children can take them safely. But if reactions occur, or if the hyperthyroidism cannot be properly controlled by these medications, or if the thyroid remains very large and unsightly, the doctor may recommend that much of the child's thyroid gland be removed surgically. Once the thyroid tissue is removed, the source of the excessive amounts of thyroid hormone is gone and the child should be cured. Indeed, thyroid surgery is usually safe and effective if the surgeon is well trained and experienced in thyroid surgery in children. Unfortunately this kind of surgery can be difficult, carrying with it the risk of damage to structures in the neck near the thyroid gland (Figure 38). A few children who are operated upon for hyperthyroidism will have surgical injury to the nerve supplying their vocal cords. Accidental removal of or damage to the nearby parathyroid glands may also occur. The former may cause a change in voice or permanent hoarseness, while the latter may produce a calcium imbalance for which the child may need to take medication for the rest of his or her life. In addition a surgical scar will result, though it usually fades and becomes less noticeable with the passage of time.

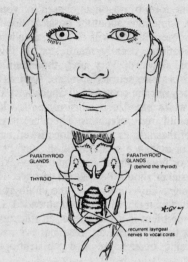

PARATHYROID
GLANDS

PARATHYROID
GLANDS
(behind the thyroid)

THYROID

recurrent layngeal
nerves to vocal cords

Figure 38 The thyroid and nearby structures in the neck.

In view of such potentially serious complications from drug and surgical treatments for hyperthyroidism in children, it would seem that physicians would choose instead to control the thyroid as we usually do in adults, by destroying some of the thyroid with radioactive iodine. Indeed this treatment is as effective as surgical removal of the thyroid and carries no risk of damage to the vocal-cord nerves or parathyroid glands. However, although it is clear that no serious complications from radioactive iodine treatment have been observed in more than forty years' experience in treating adults, physicians are aware that very young children's thyroid glands may be sensitive to the effects of radiation, and they may be more likely to develop thyroid tumors and other tumors in the years following treatment. Also, in contrast to adults, children have more years ahead of them in which to develop complications from radiation. Fortunately at this time there is no evidence that children who have been treated with radioiodine have developed any specific problems.

Radioactive iodine is an effective means of controlling

hyperthyroidism in a child, and it may prove to be as safe in children as in adults. For the time being, however, most physicians do not routinely use this treatment for children. Instead we reserve radioiodine for use in children who are allergic to antithyroid drugs or whose hyperthyroidism cannot be controlled by such drugs, and in whom thyroid surgery is not advisable or desired. You and your physician should discuss the alternatives of treatment of your child's condition carefully in an effort to understand the particular circumstances that lead to a recommendation of a specific plan of treatment.

Hyperthyroidism of the type that commonly occurs among children is a lifelong disease. It may recur at any time, and in some cases the gland may fail, resulting in hypothyroidism. Children treated surgically or with radioiodine are particularly apt to develop hypothyroidism. For these reasons any hyperthyroid child should remain under the care of a physician indefinitely. If the thyroid does fail, hypothyroidism can be treated easily with thyroid hormone replacement tablets once a day.

THE UNDERACTIVE THYROID IN INFANCY

In our country one in every four to five thousand babies is born with hypothyroidism. Here, as in most developed countries, hypothyroidism in the newborn is usually due to an absent or abnormally located and poorly functioning thyroid gland. Hypothyroidism can also be seen in infants born to mothers who took antithyroid drugs or iodine during pregnancy, either of which can pass from the mother to her baby and affect the baby's thyroid. Finally, 10 percent of the time hypothyroidism is due to one of several known inherited disorders in which the thyroid makes too little thyroid hormone as a result of a defect in the hormone-manufacturing process.

Hypothyroidism is particularly common in remote, often mountainous areas of the world where there is insufficient iodine in the diet. Iodine-deficient infants may suffer mental and physical damage from which they cannot recover even if they are eventually treated adequately with thyroid hormone. Iodine deficiency is not a problem in the United States, because our salt is iodized and iodine has been added to other foods as well.

If you have a baby born with an underactive thyroid, the baby may seem normal to you and even to the doctor who checks the infant after birth. In the next hours and days you may notice that the baby's skin has a yellowish color due to newborn *jaundice*, which clears more slowly in hypothyroid babies. It is only in the following days and weeks that the infant becomes sluggish, sleepy, and develops the hoarse cry, stuffy nose, and puffy face and body typical of the kind of hypothyroidism known as *cretinism*. But by then your baby would be at home and you might not realize at first that he or she was seriously ill. Such babies should be treated with thyroid hormone as soon as possible after birth to prevent permanent brain damage and mental retardation.

NEONATAL SCREENING FOR HYPOTHYROIDISM

Forunately if hypothyroidism due to any cause is discovered early and treated appropriately with thyroid hormone, permanent mental retardation can usually be avoided. However, it must be diagnosed as early as possible—preferably with blood tests done at birth. This is why all babies born in the United States and Canada, as well as in many other parts of the world, are now being screened for hypothyroidism at birth by means of tests done on blood obtained by heel prick or from the umbilical cord. Long-term follow-up studies have shown that hypothyroid babies who are identified early and treated within the first two months of life appear to suffer no intellectual impairment when compared with their unaffected brothers and sisters. Thus the widespread institution of neonatal-screening programs for hypothyroidism is a triumph of preventive medicine.

Finally, in addition to being certain your baby will have thyroid tests done immediately after birth, you must carefully read the labels of all medicines you take during pregnancy to be sure that they do not contain large quantities of iodine or other substances known to affect the baby. Iodized table salt poses no problem, but health foods such as kelp and some medications (for example certain cough syrups) contain large amounts of iodine. If they are taken in large quantities over a long period, they may cause not only hypothyroidism but also goiter in your baby. Obviously during pregnancy antithyroid drugs should be used in only the lowest possible dose and under the close supervision of a physician, and radioactive iodine (which might damage the baby's thyroid) should *never* be given to a pregnant woman for any reason.

HYPOTHYROIDISM IN LATER CHILDHOOD

If your child's thyroid fails after the child is six years old, the thyroid is probably affected by a low-grade inflammation known as chronic lymphocytic thyroiditis. The first sign that such a problem exists is often a painless swelling in the front of the neck caused by the enlarged thyroid. Fortunately this slight enlargement of the thyroid is usually enough to alert the pediatrician or the parents to the fact that thyroid disease is present. Since this type of thyroiditis can damage thyroid tissue and thus decrease thyroid function, symptoms and signs of hypothyroidism may follow. However, such a child may seem perfectly healthy, and the *only* evidence that the thyroid is failing may be a slowing of the growth rate. In such a case the pediatrician may be the first to suspect hypothyroidism when the child's growth rate slows and fails to keep up with the past growth pattern. Parents may have noticed symptoms of hypothyroidism long before that, including sluggishness (Figure 39), pallor, dry and itchy skin, increased sensitivity to cold, and constipation. At the same time, surprisingly, schoolwork may improve, because the child may be less active and therefore more attentive in class. Once hypothyroidism is suspected, the physician usually has no trouble in confirming the diagnosis. Blood tests will reveal a low thyroid hormone level as well as an elevated level of the pituitary thyroid stimulating hormone (TSH), described in detail in Chapter 6. Treatment of the hypothyroidism with thyroid hormone should correct the symptoms and signs of the condition, with rapid improvement in energy and mental function followed by a return to normal of the growth pattern. Do not be surprised if schoolwork suffers temporarily as the treated child becomes more aware of the environment and more involved in outside activities.

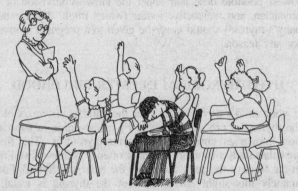

Figure 39 A hypothyroid child may be less active than normal during the day.

PAINFUL SWELLING OF THE THYROID (SUBACUTE THYROIDITIS)

Occasionally a week or two after a viral infection (often a typical sore throat), an older child may begin to complain of an unusual type of sore throat, in which the discomfort comes from a painfully swollen thyroid gland in the front of the neck. Your child may have a fever, aches, and pains and may be sick enough to stay in bed, but it is the tender goiter that suggests thyroid inflammation is present—not just a "common cold."

Blood tests will usually prove that your child's swollen thyroid is inflamed. If there is any doubt, the pediatrician may do a radioactive-thyroid uptake test, which should show no activity at all in the inflamed thyroid gland. The usual treatment is with aspirin alone, and rapid improvement is usually apparent within a day or two.

On rare occasions when the condition is severe, there may be an early period of perhaps three to four weeks during which your child may develop symptoms of hyperthyroidism due to large amounts of thyroid hormone that have leaked out of the inflamed gland. This may be followed by another three to four weeks during which your child may be sluggish from low thyroid levels until the exhausted gland begins to work again. If either of these phases is severe, the physician can prescribe medications to control symptoms, correct the thyroid hormone level, and make the child feel better. Once the disease has run its course, the child should recover completely and remain healthy.

THYROID NODULES

Thyroid nodules (lumps) that appear in childhood are usually due to thyroid inflammation (thyroiditis), benign tumors, or thyroid cysts. Fortunately thyroid nodules containing cancer are rare in children. If your child develops a thyroid cancer, it will probably be painless and the nodule or nodules will feel harder than other kinds of thyroid nodules. In addition you may notice hard and swollen lymph glands near the thyroid resulting from the spread of the cancer within the neck. As is true for most forms of cancer, prompt recognition and treatment of thyroid cancer is important, for such tumors are usually curable. If your child has or is suspected of having a thyroid nodule, you should take the child to a physician for an examination. If the physician agrees that one or more nodules are present, he or she will perform studies necessary to determine the cause of the nodule, usually including thyroid blood tests and a thyroid scan. Often a fine-needle aspiration biopsy can be performed in which a small number of cells from the nodule are obtained, which is usually enough to tell whether or not cancer is present. If cancer is found in a nodule, early treatment is imperative and should include an operation to remove as much malignant tissue as possible. Often the entire thyroid is removed, even though only a portion of the gland is affected by a malignant tumor. Removal of the whole thyroid may reduce the chance of tumor recurrence and may facilitate later follow-up and treatment. Fortunately surgery is almost always successful and complete cure is likely. As with adults who have thyroid cancer, some children will also need treatment with radioactive iodine. In addition, lifelong treatment with thyroid hormone is always given to try to prevent further growth of any cancer cells that might remain. Your child will need periodic checkups after that, since thyroid cancer may reappear even in children taking thyroid hormone medication. If that happens, additional surgery or other treatments may be required.

If your child's nodule is benign, your physician will advise you if long-term treatment to *suppress* the thyroid is indicated. The pituitary gland normally stimulates and controls the thyroid by means of TSH. Since TSH also tends to make some nodules grow, too, your physician may elect to treat your child with thyroid hormone tablets to shut off TSH production by the pituitary. Alternatively your physician may prefer to see the child periodically and not treat with thyroid hormone unless the nodule enlarges or more nodules appear.

As we said in Chapter 10, there is a rare type of thyroid cancer known as *medullary carcinoma* that tends to run in families and that can be detected by means of a blood test for *calcitonin*, a hormone made by the tumor. People with this disease tend to have tumors of other glands as well, including the adrenal glands (which can cause high blood pressure) and parathyroid glands (which can raise the blood calcium level). Children who are found to have this type of cancer have their best chance for cure if it is discovered and removed early. Therefore children in families in which this rare form of cancer has been found should have yearly calcitonin blood tests. When the tests suggest the presence of such a tumor, it should be removed at once.

SUMMARY

If your child has a thyroid problem he or she may not look or act very sick. The only evidence that thyroid trouble is present may be a change in the child's growth rate. Therefore the height and weight records that your pediatrician keeps often prove helpful in detecting thyroid disease. The treatments we use for thyroid disorders, including thyroid hormone, antithyroid drugs, radioactive iodine, and thyroid surgery, are effective and almost always curative. Some of these treatments have side effects that could be serious for some children. However, even though there may not be one "best" treatment for your child's thyroid problem, it should be possible for you as a parent to understand why your child's physician recommends a particular way of treating that condition. The authors hope this chapter will help you to communicate more effectively with your child's physician.

CHAPTER THIRTEEN

Thyroid Trouble During and Following Pregnancy

> I have in five cases seen coincident ... enlargement of the heart and ... of the thyroid gland. The first case ... was that of Grace B., a married woman, aged thirty seven, in the month of August, 1786. About three months after lying-in, while she was suckling her child, a lump of about the size of a walnut was perceived on the right side of her neck. This continued to enlarge till ... it occupied both sides of her neck. The part that swelled was the thyroid gland. ... The eyes were protruded from their sockets, and the countenance exhibited an appearance of agitation and distress.
>
> —From *Collections from the Unpublished Medical Writings of Caleb Hillier Parry*. London: Underwoods. 1825; 2: 111.

THE THYROID DURING PREGNANCY

If you are pregnant, the changes that are happening in your body because of the pregnancy may make it difficult for both you and your physician to tell if something is happening to your thyroid, as well. For example an overactive thyroid may make you feel nervous, overheated, shaky, and flushed—any of which may happen to a woman in normal pregnancy who has a healthy thyroid. Furthermore since your physician must consider the baby inside you, the thyroid tests and treatment for you will be different from what they would be if you were not pregnant. Despite these difficulties, if you do develop a problem with your thyroid gland during pregnancy, it can be diagnosed correctly and treated successfully.

Increased amounts of female sex hormones circulate in your blood during pregnancy, causing your blood level of thyroid hormone to rise. However, although the total amount of thyroid hormone is increased, almost all of the extra thyroid hormone is in an inactive condition bound to

164

certain proteins in your blood and therefore has no effect on you or your unborn child. Recent research has shown that there may be a slight increase in your free or active thyroid-hormone level in the first three months of pregnancy, and a slight decrease in the last three months, but no evidence has been found that these mild changes cause risks to normal women or their children.

The mild hyperthyroidism in early pregnancy develops due to increased levels of a placental hormone known as *human chorionic gonadotropin*, or *HCG*, which cause the thyroid gland to increase production of thyroid hormones. This is the hormone that your physician measures to diagnose pregnancy. These changes may cause your thyroid to become a little larger, but this is rarely noticeable in a normal woman unless she lives in a country in which dietary iodine deficiency provides an additional stimulus toward thyroid growth. So if you live in the United States or Canada, where there is plenty of iodine in your diet, and develop a goiter during pregnancy, it is likely that you have a thyroid problem. In that case your obstetrician will probably arrange for you to have thyroid tests performed. Alternatively you may be referred to a specialist for a thyroid evaluation.

The Overactive Thyroid in Pregnancy

Hyperthyroidism occurs in only about one out of every five hundred pregnant women. Hyperthyroid women often do not have normal reproductive cycles and therefore have difficulty both in becoming pregnant and in maintaining a normal pregnancy. However, if you do have an overactive thyroid that remains markedly overactive throughout your pregnancy, there are increased health risks for you as well as your baby. You may experience heart complications including heart-rhythm problems and heart failure, and your baby is more likely to be premature and small than if your thyroid were normal. On the other hand, if your thyroid is only slightly overactive, or if it can be controlled during pregnancy, there is no added risk to you and little, if any, danger to your baby.

Hyperthyroidism can be difficult to recognize in pregnancy, since many of the symptoms and signs of hyperthyroidism occur in normal pregnancy. Pregnant women may normally experience a fast pulse, nervousness, heat intolerance, flushing, and increased perspiration. Hyperthyroidism therefore may seem like no more than an exaggeration of these "normal" signs of a healthy pregnancy. Usually, however, there are other clues that the thyroid is overactive. Your heart rate may be especially fast—more than 120 beats per minute. You may fail to gain weight, and may even lose weight as calories are burned up at a rapid rate. You may experience marked muscular weakness, and elevated eyelids may make your eyes seem bigger. Finally, your thyroid may grow larger as it becomes overactive.

If your obstetrician suspects that you have hyperthyroidism, it is usually easy to diagnose by means of blood tests that show decreased or undetectable levels of thyroid–stimulating hormone (TSH) and increased levels of active (free) thyroid hormone. Radioactive iodine cannot be used as a further test for hyperthyroidism if you are pregnant because it would be passed from your body across the placenta to your baby and might damage its thyroid tissue. If the diagnosis is in doubt, your obstetrician may simply wait and repeat thyroid blood tests a few weeks later, since a mild degree of hyperthyroidism does not appear to pose a significant danger to either you or your unborn child.

Two antithyroid drugs may be used to treat hyperthyroidism: propylthiouracil (PTU) and methimazole (Tapazole), both of which block the manufacture of thyroid hormone by the thyroid gland. Most physicians prefer to use PTU in pregnancy. Far less PTU than methimazole crosses your placenta to the baby, so there is less chance of the baby becoming hypothyroid or developing a goiter during pregnancy. Since both of these drugs can cross from your system into your baby's blood stream and may affect your baby's thyroid function, your treatment dosage must be kept to a minimum. At first enough of the drug must be given to bring your hyperthyroidism under control. As soon as that control has been achieved, however, the dosage is reduced to the lowest possible amount that will keep you healthy and yet minimize the drug effect on your unborn child. In practice this usually means a total daily dose of less than 200 milligrams of PTV or 20 milligrams of methimazole, though sometimes it is possible to reduce the amount of antithyroid drug even further in the later stages of pregnancy, when hyperthyroidism often becomes milder.

Some patients taking PTV or methimazole may become allergic to these drugs and develop a red skin rash, itching, or hives. More rarely these drugs can cause a dangerous decrease in certain white blood cells (neutrophils) that normally help control infections. Therefore if you are taking one of these drugs and develop a rash, itching, hives, or evidence of an infection (such as a fever or sore throat), you should immediately stop the drug and contact your physician that day. If you have a fever or sore throat, you will need to have a blood test to be sure that an infection has not developed due to a lowering of your white cell count. If the neutrophil count is normal and there is no evidence of drug allergy, your physician will probably restart your antithyroid drug even while you are being treated for the infection. If, on the other hand, your neutrophil count is low, or your physician finds other evidence of drug allergy, another form of treatment for your hyperthyroidism must be chosen.

Propranolol (Inderal) and other so-called beta-blockers, which block the action of thyroid hormone on the body, may be used in pregnancy for short periods of time to help control symptoms of hyperthyroidism. These drugs are extremely successful in slowing a fast pulse rate and reducing nervousness and anxiety, but have unfortunate side effects that keep us from using them for a long period of time during pregnancy. Propranolol and similar drugs may slow the growth and development of your unborn baby. Furthermore some medical reports suggest that if you are taking one of these drugs at the end of pregnancy, your baby may be born with difficulty breathing, a slow pulse, and low blood sugar. For these reasons we prefer to use propranolol and other beta-blockers only briefly and early in pregnancy, and then only if the hyperthyroidism is severe.

In some instances a physician will recommend an operation to remove your thyroid gland as a way of treating hyperthyroidism when you are pregnant. If so, the surgery will usually be delayed until after the third month of pregnancy, because any kind of surgery earlier in pregnancy is associated with a slightly increased risk of miscarriage. A few weeks' treatment with an antithyroid drug or a few days' treatment with the thyroid-hormone-blocking drug propranolol are usually given to control the overactive thyroid before your thyroid operation is performed. Iodine, which might ordinarily be prescribed, is not usually used to prepare a pregnant woman for thyroid surgery, since it could affect the baby's thyroid too. In like manner *radioactive iodine* cannot be used to treat hyperthyroidism during pregnancy, for the radioiodine would cross from you into your baby and damage the baby's thyroid.

If you have been hyperthyroid during your pregnancy (or at anytime earlier in your life), your doctor will examine your baby for *neonatal hyperthyroidism.* This condition may occur if the thyroid stimulating antibodies that cause your own thyroid to be overactive cross the placenta to your unborn baby in large enough quantities to stimulate your baby's thyroid to overactivity. Fortunately this condition is extremely rare and develops in only about one in every seventy babies born to hyperthyroid mothers. If such a condition is found, it is usually mild, requires no treatment, and subsides in a few weeks. If it is severe, however, it may cause thyroid enlargement and make the infant sick with marked irritability and a very rapid heartbeat, and may interfere with the baby's growth in the first days and weeks of life. If so, the baby's thyroid overactivity can be controlled with medication until it subsides (see Chapter 12).

If you took antithyroid drugs during pregnancy, the doctors will also examine your baby for evidence of an underactive thyroid (hypothyroidism) and thyroid enlargement (goiter). If either condition has been caused by your medications, treatment is not usually required since the problem will rapidly disappear as these drugs leave your baby's body.

On the other hand, one in every four to five thousand babies is born with hypothyroidism due to an underlying thyroid problem of its own. That kind of hypothyroidism will not go away by itself and therefore must be recognized and treated as early as possible. Fortunately thyroid tests are now performed on all newborn babies in this country, so these disorders are almost always found and successfully treated before permanent harm is done.

If you have been hyperthyroid during a pregnancy, your thyroid condition should be carefully watched in the weeks following the birth of your baby. Your thyroid may gradually become more overactive following delivery. If so, and if you are breast-feeding your baby, your physician must still consider your baby's welfare in deciding how to continue to best treat your thyroid. It is generally advised that if you are breast-feeing, you should not take the antithyroid drugs PTV or methimazole, since both appear in breast milk. Once ingested by the baby, it is possible they will interfere with your infant's thyroid gland. However, the amounts of these drugs that get into breast milk are very small, and probably pose little risk to the child. This is especially true for PTV. So if you strongly desire to nurse while taking this drug, you may do so, but close monitoring of your infant's thyroid-hormone levels and white blood cell count is essential.

It is imperative that you not be treated for hyperthyroidism with radioactive iodine while you are breast-feeding, for in such a case some of the radioactive iodine would be passed on to your baby in your milk. The amount of radioactive iodine that your baby would receive in this manner might cause subsequent harm to his or her thyroid. Therefore if you are breast-feeing and must be given radioactive iodine to control an overactive thyroid, you will find that your physician will ask you to stop breast-feeding before the treatment is given and until the radioactivity has disappeared from your milk. This may take many weeks, and it is likely that breast-feeding will have to be discontinued altogether.

The Underactive Thyroid in Pregnancy

If your physician suspects that you have an underactive thyroid, he or she will measure your blood level of thyroid-stimulating hormone (TSH) as well as your blood level of thyroid hormone. Since the elevated levels of sex hormones that occur in pregnancy cause the thyroid hormone level to rise, it is possible for a pregnant woman with an *underactive* thyroid to have what seems to be a normal blood level of thyroid hormone, which could cause an error or delay in the discovery of a thyroid deficiency. But although the total thyroid-hormone level is normal, the "free" or "unbound" level is below normal. (See Chapter 1 for a more complete discussion of this point.) Fortunately an elevation of TSH is the most reliable indication of an underactive thyroid.

If you are found to have hypothyroidism while you are pregnant, your physician should treat you promptly with thyroid hormone to avoid possible complications. Although rare, these include increased miscarriage, high blood pressure, bleeding after pregnancy, and abnormal development in the baby after pregnancy.

If you have been previously diagnosed with hypothyroidism before you became pregnant, you should be aware that your dose of thyroid hormone may need to be increased during your pregnancy. Blood tests to evaluate the adequacy of your thyroid dose should be performed periodically through the pregnancy because the amount of thyroid hormone you need may continue to rise. After delivery, your thyroid prescription should be cut back to or near your original dose.

Until recently doctors believed that children born to mothers who were hypothyroid in early pregnancy were at high risk for decreased intelligence. However, more recent studies have found normal intelligence in a number of these children. Complications are probably more likely if the hypothyroidism is severe, but do occur occasionally even when maternal hypothyroidism is mild. Therefore your physician should treat even mild hypothyroidism as soon as the condition is recognized to minimize the possibility of such problems. Frequent measurements of free T4 and TSH blood levels will allow your doctor to know when your thyroid dosage is adequate.

Thyroid Nodules in Pregnancy

Thyroid lumps or nodules in pregnancy present a special problem because radioactive iodine scans cannot be used as a way of evaluating their function. The radioactive iodine used in such scanning procedures would be a risk to your unborn child, whose thyroid might be damaged even by a low dose of radioiodine. Actually the baby's thyroid doesn't take up iodine until about the tenth week of pregnancy, but any radiation exposure to the fetus should be avoided if possible.

If you do develop a thyroid nodule during pregnancy, other tests can be done that will tell why the nodule has developed and yet will not endanger you or your child. Thyroid blood tests can indicate whether your nodule is associated with a more general condition, such as an overactive or underactive thyroid. A thyroid ultrasound test can be used to tell whether a nodule is solid or is a fluid-filled cyst. Most important, a fine-needle biopsy can be performed with complete safety during the pregnancy, and an examination of the tissue obtained should reveal the cause of the nodule.

If a biopsy shows that your thyroid nodule is harmless, it can be left alone or treated with thyroid hormone. If the nodule is found to contain cancer, it can be removed in an operation, preferably after the third month of the pregnancy, when there is the least risk to your baby from any surgical procedure. Alternatively thyroid-hormone treatment can be given to help control the cancer, just as in a nonpregnant patient, and surgery can be performed after delivery.

In summary, if you have a thyroid problem during pregnancy, it can be diagnosed and treated effectively even though the hormonal changes that occur in pregnancy may alter your thyroid blood tests to some degree. The treatment of your thyroid condition in pregnancy is similar to that given to nonpregnant women, though in some situations treatment may be modified to avoid endangering your unborn child. When the baby is born, he or she will be carefully examined for evidence of a thyroid problem and will have a thyroid blood test performed as a routine measure.

THYROID DYSFUNCTION AFTER PREGNANCY

A mother's immune system appears to be suppressed during pregnancy as a protection for her baby, who, after all, could be considered a foreign invader. In the months after delivery, however, autoimmune activity in the mother tends to increase.

Graves' Disease

If you had Graves' disease in the early stages of pregnancy, it is possible that your immune system was suppressed as your pregnancy progressed. Thus the severity of your hyperthyroidism may have diminished and you felt better. It is even possible that you stopped needing any medication. If that is your situation, your physician will likely observe your condition carefully in the months after you deliver, because when your immune system becomes active, you may well become hyperthyroid again. Even if you have never been hyperthyroid before, this postpartum period is one of the more common times for Graves' disease to begin. Your increased immune activity may induce antibody activity that can trigger Graves' disease if you have the tendency to this autoimmune disorder.

Although the symptoms may be mild and hard to evaluate in the new mother, palpitations, nervousness, and emotional ups and downs may suggest the condition. You may notice a swelling in your neck due to an enlarged thyroid gland. Your physician may confirm the diagnosis by blood tests that show increased levels of thyroid hormones and a low or undetectable level of TSH.

A radioactive-iodine uptake test should only be performed in women who are not breast-feeding or who are willing to stop nursing until the radioiodine disappears from their milk. Usually breast feeding can be resumed in one to two days if the short-lived ^{123}I isotope of radioactive iodine or radioactive technetium is used. This test is extremely helpful in differentiating hyperthyroidism due to Graves' disease (in which the uptake of iodine by the thyroid is increased) from that due to thyroiditis (in which there should be little or no uptake by the inflamed thyroid). As you will see, the treatments for the two conditions are quite different.

If you have Graves' disease, your treatment possibilities are the same as those of any patient with this condition, though your physician will have special requirements if you are nursing your baby. Antithyroid drugs (PTU and methimazole) can be carried to your baby in breast milk, so your physician may want to monitor the baby's thyroid function if such treatment is prolonged.

The radioiodine isotope ^{131}I used to treat hyperthyroidism has a longer half-life in the body than the ^{123}I isotope employed in thyroid testing. Therefore if your physician decides that radioactive iodine is the best treatment for you, there will be important restrictions you will need to understand. You will probably have to stop nursing, because the radioactive iodine from a treatment dose of ^{131}I remains in your body and breast milk for up to two months. You will also have to limit your contact with your baby, especially in the first week after treatment, to avoid exposing your child to unnecessary radiation.

Surgery is an alternative treatment. Though it has added risks (see Chapter 5), your physician may have special reasons for recommending it for you.

If these precautions are followed, your Graves' disease should be easily controlled and you can expect a return to good health within two or three months.

Postpartum Thyroiditis

If you experience thyroid dysfunction in the postpartum period, it is quite possible that you do not have Graves' disease. It is more likely that your problem is thyroiditis, an inflammation of the thyroid gland due to antibodies made by your immune system (see Chapter 3).

Investigations in different parts of the world have found the incidence of postpartum thyroiditis to vary from 3 to 21 percent of all women who become pregnant.* Such a wide range is likely a result of differences in dietary iodine levels, the timing of thyroid testing, and the sensitivity of testing methods. Studies in the United States suggest a fre-

---

*A recent review of several patient surveys suggests that in the United States thyroid dysfunction occurs after 4.9 percent of all pregnancies: 2.2 percent become hypothyroid; 1.7 percent hyperthyroid; and 1 percent hyperthyroid then hypothyroid. A small percentage of the second group (0.2 percent of the total) develop Graves' disease. Gerstein HC. How common is postpartum thyroiditis? *Archives of Internal Medicine.* 1990; 150: 1397.

quency of about 5 to 8 percent, but with a much higher rate among individuals who have evidence of a tendency to develop autoimmune disorders. Thus the chance of thyroid dysfunction after pregnancy for women who have a positive blood test for antithyroid antibodies increases to about 50 percent.

Your thyroid gland is a reservoir that stores large amounts of thyroid hormone. Under normal circumstances the release of this hormone is carefully regulated to meet your body's needs. When the thyroid becomes inflamed in postpartum thyroiditis, damage to the cells may release large quantities of hormones into your blood stream, which can result in hyperthyroidism that may last for one to three months. If that happens to you, you may feel fine as long as the rise in your hormone levels is moderate. On the other hand you may become anxious and experience tremors, palpitations, and muscle weakness if your hormone levels increase dramatically or if some other medical condition makes you particularly sensitive to the hormone change. If you are one of the few patients who develops symptoms while you are hyperthyroid, your physician may prescribe a beta-adrenergic blocking drug such as propranolol or atenolol to slow your rapid pulse and calm your anxiety.

As shown in figure 40, after two or three months of postpartum hyperthyroidism, one of three things will happen. If

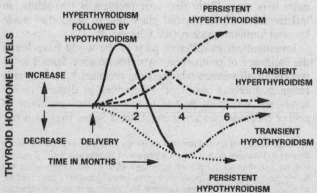

Figure 40 Thyroid dysfunction after pregnancy.

you have developed Graves' disease, you may remain hyperthyroid. Alternatively your thyroid hormone levels may return to normal, and you may recover (transient hyperthyroidism). Finally, if your thyroid tissues have been severely damaged by the inflammatory process, your gland may not heal so readily. In this case once the stores of thyroid hormones have been exhausted, you may become hypothyroid. At this point you may feel tired, cold, and depressed, and experience muscle cramps and constipation, but these symptoms should improve with thyroid hormone treatment. This hypothyroid period commonly lasts about three to six months, after which the gland should recover and start manufacturing and releasing thyroid hormones once again.

About twenty-five percent of patients do remain permanently hypothyroid and require lifelong treatment, while in others thyroid dysfunction may return after another pregnancy or in later years. At a minimum your physician will want to perform an annual TSH blood test to assess your thyroid function.

SUMMARY

If a thyroid problem develops during or after pregnancy, it can be diagnosed even though the hormonal changes that occur in pregnancy may alter your thyroid tests. The treatment of a thyroid condition before or after pregnancy is similar to that given to nonpregnant women, though in some situations it may be modified to avoid endangering your unborn child or baby. When your baby is born, he or she will be carefully examined for evidence of a thyroid problem and will have a thyroid blood test performed as a routine measure.

CHAPTER FOURTEEN

Thyroid Problems in Older Individuals

> Here are two very distinctly different types of hyperthyroidism and so atypical may be the so-called apathetic hyperthyroidism without its eye signs, without goiter, without striking tachycardia, and striking heart action, with low basal rates, without obvious activation reaction, the diagnosis is not infrequently overlooked through long periods of time.
>
> —Lahey FH. Non-activated (apathetic) types of hyperthyroidism. *New England Journal of Medicine.* 1931; 204: 747.

If you are over sixty-five and develop a thyroid problem, it is more likely to go unrecognized than if you were twenty or thirty years younger. This is because the symptoms and signs of hyper- and hypothyroidism for an elderly patient are often very subtle and different from those in a younger person. The physical changes in your body as you have gotten older can alter the way thyroid hormones affect you.

It is also possible that you have a new family physician. Your former doctor may have retired, or you may have moved. If so, your new doctor may not know you as well and may miss the subtle changes caused by a new thyroid problem.

HYPERTHYROIDISM

Approximately 15 percent of all thyrotoxic patients are over the age of sixty. Several population surveys suggest a prevalence of hyperthyroidism in this age group from 0.5 to 2.5 percent. In many individuals the symptoms are typical and include hyperactivity, palpitations, tremor, and weight loss despite a good appetite. However, the signs of an overactive thyroid, especially if they are minor, may be simply accepted as the natural characteristics of aging. Thus nervousness, weakness, and a gradual decline in weight with a poor appetite may not suggest hyperthyroidism to a physician, caretaker, or even a close relative. For example older persons often have problems with heart palpitations or heart pain known as angina as their thyroid becomes overactive. But these symptoms may be accepted as inevitable characteristics of an older heart rather than clues to a new thyroid problem. Furthermore the thyroid gland of an older individual may not enlarge when it becomes overactive.

All of these symptoms suggest the need for a general checkup, but a TSH blood test should be included in the evaluation.

Simple Diagnosis

Once suspected, the diagnosis of hyperthyroidism should be just as straightforward as in a younger person. A blood test will show that the concentration of TSH is low or absent while thyroid-hormone levels are increased. If the radioactive-iodine uptake is increased and a thyroid scan shows diffuse uptake of iodine throughout the gland, the problem is Graves' disease. A scan showing one or more isolated areas of activity indicates that the problem is a toxic nodular goiter, or Plummer's disease.

Important Differences in Treatment

Your physician will probably be very careful in treating hyperthyroidism that develops late in life, because underlying heart problems could be worsened by further increases in thyroid-hormone levels. It is not uncommon for a physician simply to treat a hyperthyroid younger person with radioactive iodine while controlling symptoms such as a rapid pulse with a *beta-adrenergic blocking drug* such as *atenolol* or *propranolol*. In an older individual, however, physicians tend to be more cautious about using radioactive iodine, since this treatment may be associated with a temporary increase in thyroid hormone levels, which could induce arrhythmia or angina. Therefore your physician may choose to begin treatment with an antithyroid drug (PTV or

Tapazole). After four to six weeks these drugs should have decreased your thyroid hormone levels to normal. At that point your physician can stop the antithyroid drug and treat you a few days later with radioactive iodine. If your thyroid hormone levels increase again during the two to three months it takes the radioiodine to control your overactive thyroid permanently, your physician may temporarily restart the antithyroid drug or prescribe a beta-adrenergic blocking drug to control thyroid function and prevent cardiac complications.

HYPOTHYROIDISM

Hypothyroidism may be even more difficult to recognize in an older person, but is more common than hyperthyroidism in the elderly. Investigators in the large, ongoing population survey known as the Framingham Study have reported that by age sixty, 16.9 percent of women and 8.2 percent of men have evidence of a failing thyroid as manifested by an increased blood level of thyroid stimulating hormone (TSH). Other studies from around the world have shown that many of these individuals progress to actual hypothyroidism.

As with hyperthyroidism, the symptoms of a failing thyroid may be subtle and easily overlooked in an older person. We expect some fatigue, chilliness, constipation, forgetfulness, muscle cramps, hair loss, and depression as we get older, but they may actually be signs of a failing thyroid.

Straightforward Diagnosis

When hypothyroidism is suspected, a TSH blood test is usually all that is necessary to confirm the diagnosis. The concentration of TSH will increase as the pituitary tries to stimulate the failing thyroid. If the TSH is increased, your physician may also measure thyroid hormone levels to obtain information about the degree of thyroid deficiency to help determine the amount of thyroid hormone that will be required in treatment.

Thyroid Treatment: Start Low and Increase Slowly

Because of the possibility of underlying heart disease, your physician will probably start to treat your thyroid deficiency with a very low dose of thyroxine. It is not uncommon to begin with just 25 micrograms every other day, with gradual monthly increases in dose until your TSH level is normal. Even patients with angina or heart rhythm problems can usually tolerate such a schedule, and the majority exhibit an improved cardiac condition as thyroid levels move toward normal.

THYROID NODULES AND CANCER

The older you get, the more likely you are to have a thyroid nodule. Many of these are tiny and thus are rarely noticed in the course of a standard health examination, and fortunately very few contain cancer. But if your physician does discover a lump in your thyroid, he or she may suggest an evaluation with thyroid-hormone and TSH-blood tests and a radioactive-iodine thyroid scan. If your nodule concentrates iodine normally in the scan image, your physician will probably be satisfied that the lump is harmless and simply reexamine your neck and run a new TSH test to look for hypothyroidism at regular follow-up visits.

If the nodule does not concentrate radioiodine in the thyroid scan, your physician may recommend a fine-needle biopsy to be sure that it does not contain cancer. If the biopsy specimen reveals cancer cells, the nodule should be removed, and additional treatment with radioactive iodine may be indicated. Fortunately these treatments do not normally present a significant risk for an older individual, and usually cure the condition. (See Chapter 10 for a more complete description of the evaluation and treatment of thyroid nodules.)

SUMMARY

Thyroid conditions are usually easily identified and treated in older individuals once the diagnosis is suspected. The problem is that thyroid conditions can go unrecognized due to their gradual and subtle onset or because such symptoms are accepted as a normal manifestation of getting old.

We recommend that a thyroid examination and an occasional TSH blood test be part of a regular checkup for any woman over fifty and men and women over the age of sixty, and especially if someone in the family has had a thyroid problem or a related autoimmune condition. Such individuals should also have occasional blood tests measuring the level of vitamin B12. Deficiencies of vitamin B12 are common in thyroid families and are often difficult to recognize, yet they can cause anemia and neurological or mental changes that can be treated and often cured by treatment with the vitamin (see Chapter 9).

Finally, if you are a young person with a thyroid or related autoimmune disorder, looking for these indicators may help you recognize thyroid problems among your older relatives.

CHAPTER FIFTEEN

Drugs, Food, Stress, Emotions, and Your Thyroid

A person develops exophthalmic goiter after a fright because he is a special type of person. Another might develop asthma or peptic ulcer or manic depressive psychosis after an identical experience. Many more would develop nothing more than very temporary "jitters." We must look upon the development of exophthalmic goiter after psychic trauma as the result of a stimulus applied to an individual preconditioned to make that remarkable response. The patient is a loaded gun. The psychic trauma pulls the trigger.

—Means JH. *The Thyroid and Its Diseases*
New York: J. B. Lippincott Co. 1937: 565.

DRUGS

Iodine

Iodine is the cause of more thyroid problems than all other food substances combined. You can get sick from eating either too much or too little iodine. In a few countries, especially in remote mountainous areas where the daily iodine intake is less than 25 micrograms per day, we find the most severe forms of hypothyroidism, including *cretinism*. This tragic disorder results from extreme iodine deficiency—affected children are born with such marked mental and physical retardation, including deaf-mutism and dwarfism, that they can never be productive members of society. The worldwide problem of iodine deficiency is much larger and extremely serious. One billion people (one-fifth of the world's population) do not get enough iodine in their diets, and countless population studies have shown that they have thyroid-related problems. In addition to unsightly goiters, they experience increased infant mortality, infertility, impaired growth, and frequent or "endemic" hypothyroidism. Most harmful are the widespread milder forms of developmental retardation that cause poor performance in school and in the workplace. These factors are reflected in impaired social and economic development. In fact iodine deficiency is the leading cause of preventable mental deficiency in the world today.

The world map (Figure 41) shows that iodine deficiency is found almost everywhere in the world except North America. The state of dietary iodine in the former Soviet Union is not well known. However, there are some data that suggest that lack of iodine is common in some areas and may have worsened the effect of the Chernobyl accident on inhabitants of that region. Lacking normal amounts of dietary iodine, their thyroid glands absorbed more radioactive iodine from fallout and thus increased their subsequent risks for thyroid failure and thyroid cancer.

THE WORLD

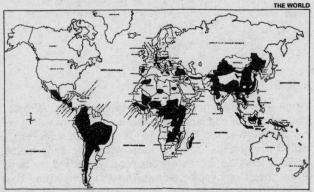

Figure 41   The world's iodine-deficient regions.

An important international effort is now under way to eradicate iodine deficiency worldwide by the year 2000. Led by the International Council for the Control of Iodine Deficiency Disorders (ICCIDD), such agencies as UNICEF, the World Health Organization, the World Bank, and the Thyroid Foundation of America (TFA) are supporting programs to correct iodine deficiency by adding iodine to salt and city water supplies and by individual treatments such as the administration of iodized oil orally or by injection. Here is a wonderful opportunity for you to help a most worthy cause. For more information, contact the ICCIDD or TFA at the addresses or telephone numbers listed in Appendix 7.

In contrast, inhabitants of the United States, Canada, Japan, and certain other countries eat more iodine than is really necessary. The Food and Nutrition Board of the National Research Council has recommended a daily intake of 150 to 300 micrograms of iodine per day. If you live in the United States, your daily dietary intake is probably between 200 and 700 micrograms per day, because extra iodine has been added to bread, milk, salt, and other foods that you frequently consume.

In countries where seaweed, such as *dulse*, is eaten, the consumption of iodine may be much higher. One study found that the inhabitants of the Japanese island of Hokkaido, who consume large quantities of a seaweed called *kombu*, take in more than 200 milligrams (200,000 micrograms) of iodine per day, a thousand times the recommended daily requirement. Although there is a 10 percent incidence of thyroid enlargement or goiter on Hokkaido, the inhabitants do not appear to have an increased risk for other thyroid problems.

TABLE 4

The Effect of Alteration in Dietary Iodine Intake

Recommended Range of Daily Iodine Intake:
150–300 micrograms*/day
Actual Range of Daily Iodine Intake—U.S.A.:
200–700 micrograms/day

ILLNESS CAUSED BY ALTERED IODINE INTAKE

TOO LITTLE IODINE	
Less than 25 micrograms Iodine/day	Some children born with goiter, hypothyroidism, retardation, cretinism.
Less than 50 micrograms Iodine/day	Goiter in some adults.

TOO MUCH IODINE

Approximately 1 milligram daily	May cause *hyperthyroidism* in elderly people who have nodular goiters.
Approximately 10 milligrams daily	Some babies born with *goiter* if mother takes this much iodine during pregnancy.
Approximately 20 milligrams daily	Some people with Graves' disease can become *hypothyroid*—more likely if they have had radioiodine treatment or surgical removal of part of their thyroid in the past.
Approximately 200 milligrams daily	Healthy people: slight change in thyroid hormone level but still feel well. Newborn babies: may be *hypothyroid* at birth. People with Hashimoto's disease (chronic thyroiditis): 50 percent become *hypothyroid*. Patient with Graves' disease (diffuse toxic goiter): *hypothyroidism* common, especially in those previously treated with radioiodine or a thyroid operation. Patients with nodular goiter: 50 percent become *hyperthyroid* (some do so on much less iodine—see above).

*1000 micrograms = 1 milligram
  1000 milligrams = 1 gram
     28.4 grams = 1 ounce
**One kelp tablet usually contains 150 micrograms of iodine.
  5 drops of "Saturated Solution of Potassium Iodide" (given as an expectorant) contain 180 milligrams of iodine.
  A kidney X ray (IVP) gives you 10–20 grams of iodine.
  A gall bladder X ray (cholecystogram) gives about 2 grams of iodine.
  Other iodine-containing medications include Quadrinal, Ornade, and Organidin used for coughs and colds, Combid given for stomach problems, and Amiodarone, which is prescribed for some heart patients. Many vitamin-mineral preparations also contain 150–300 micrograms of iodine per capsule—a potential danger for those who take them in large amounts.

Normal individuals seem to have the ability to control the amount of iodine that actually enters their thyroid gland even if their diet is supplemented with extra iodine. However, as shown in Table 4, if you have a problem with your thyroid, you may be more likely to develop a change in thyroid function if you ingest too much iodine either in your diet or in other ways. That would be true, for example, if you ever had hyperthyroidism due to a generalized overactivity of your thyroid gland (diffuse toxic goiter or Graves' disease) or if you have a low-grade inflammation of your thyroid known as chronic lymphocytic thyroiditis (Hashimoto's disease). Either condition would give you a tendency to develop hypothyroidism if you were exposed to even a modest amount of extra iodine. In fact patients who have had Graves' disease have become hypothyroid after ingesting as little as 18 milligrams of iodine per day.

Unborn babies are also very sensitive to iodine excess. Therefore if you are pregnant and ingest large quantities of iodine in the form of a medication, kelp, or another form of seaweed, you risk having your baby born with a goiter and possibly with an underactive thyroid as well. A large goiter could compress the baby's windpipe and interfere with breathing. Moreover since iodine can also be transmitted from mother to child in breast milk, you should avoid health foods and medications that contain extra iodine while nursing your baby.

An abrupt increase in dietary iodine can cause *hyper*thyroidism in people living in iodine-deficient areas of the world. Epidemics of hyperthyroidism have been seen in several countries when iodine was added to the national diet to correct a long-standing problem of widespread iodine deficiency. This happened in the United States in the 1920s, when health authorities added iodine to salt.

Hyperthyroidism caused by excess iodine also has been observed in the United States and other parts of the world where dietary iodine is sufficient. In such areas older patients with lumpy thyroids (nodular goiters) are those most likely to be affected by an increase in iodine intake. They are more likely to have complications from the rapid pulse or irregular heart rhythm that may happen when their thyroid becomes overactive.

Therefore if you have Graves' or Hashimoto's disease, are pregnant or nursing a baby, or if you have a nodular goiter, you should try to avoid an abrupt increase in your iodine intake. Do *not* eat kelp, and do read labels on bottles of vitamins and other medications. If you are having an X ray for which a dye is given to you by mouth or by injection, find out if there is iodine in it. This is likely if the X ray is of your kidney, spinal canal, gall bladder, or blood vessels. This is not to say you cannot take a medication that contains iodine or that you shouldn't have one of these special X rays. Rather, if that is your situation, your doctor may choose to examine you after you take the medication or have the X ray to be sure that your thyroid function has not changed.

The natural iodine content of most foods is low. It is highest in seafoods, and there are variable amounts in bread, milk, eggs, and meat. Fruits contain little iodine, as do vegetables, with the exception of spinach. The exact amounts of iodine in these foodstuffs vary so widely and depend on so many factors that it is no longer possible to make a satisfactory list of the iodine content of foods. Instead the message here is to eat a "regular diet" during pregnancy and while breast feeding or if you know you have a thyroid condition. You do not need to avoid iodized salt, bread, and seafood—just don't take in extra iodine if possible in special foods, such as kelp.

Some medications that contain a lot of iodine are important treatments for critical problems. A good example is the heart drug *amiodarone*, which physicians are using increasingly to stabilize life-threatening heart-rhythm problems. Each tablet contains 75 milligrams of iodine, and the average person taking the drug gets about 9 milligrams of extra iodine released into his or her bloodstream every day. If you live in the United States and need to take amiodarone, you have about a 20 percent chance of developing hypothyroidism, and a slight risk for hyperthyroidism. Since such a change in thyroid function may not occur immediately, your physician will likely check your thyroid periodically with a TSH blood test. Similarly other foods or necessary medications can be used under your doctor's supervision.

If you or your physician wants to know more about your

iodine intake, the best thing to do is to measure the iodine content of your urine. In a general way the amount of iodine in your urine is equal to the amount you take in from all sources, including food, medications, and special X-ray dyes. Such a test could be helpful if you are pregnant and want to know exactly how much iodine you are taking in. However, in most cases that information is far less important than a measurement of your thyroid hormone and TSH blood levels.

Lithium

Lithium is a drug that is being used increasingly (and quite effectively) to treat certain types of mental illness, especially *bipolar disease*, the up-and-down mood swings also known as *manic-depressive* illness. Lithium has been shown to affect thyroid gland function and size in some patients. In addition to inhibiting the manufacture of thyroid hormones, lithium may cause immune damage to thyroid cells similar to that caused by chronic thyroiditis. The same patients who get goiter and hypothyroidism from iodine— those with a history of hyperthyroidism due to Graves' disease and thyroiditis due to Hashimoto's disease—are also those most likely to have these problems from lithium. However, even if you have Graves' or Hashimoto's disease, you can still take lithium safely. If you need to take lithium, your physician may choose to test your blood for anti-thyroid antibodies. If the test is positive, according to one study, you have a 30 percent chance of developing hypothyroidism in the next eight months. But whether or not you have an antibody test, your doctor will probably examine your thyroid and check your thyroid hormone (T4) and TSH level periodically while you are on the drug. If thyroid deficiency is found, you do not need to stop lithium, for supplemental thyroid hormone administration can correct your deficiency and permit you to continue to take this useful drug.

Selenium

Recently a lack of the trace element *selenium* has been shown to be another rare cause of thyroid dysfunction. In a remote part of Zaire, inhabitants deficient in both iodine and selenium are at risk not only for goiter but also for severe thyroid failure and cretinism. Selenium is normally found in everyone's thyroid gland and protects against a buildup of certain potentially toxic chemicals including hydrogen peroxide. Without selenium the effects of iodine deficiency are much more serious.

Drugs That May Affect Thyroid-Hormone Binding

In Chapter 2 we described the way most thyroid hormones travel in your bloodstream bound to proteins. These bound hormones do not actively affect your body. Certain drugs can change thyroid hormone binding and thus alter thyroid blood tests, even though they don't affect the amounts of free or active hormones that are working in your body. Female hormones (estrogens) can increase binding; male hormones (androgens) and Dilantin are commonly used drugs that may decrease binding. The former increases the total amounts of T4 and T3 in your blood while the latter decrease the concentrations of these hormones. Since the amount of free or active hormone remains the same in either case, you feel fine. If you take one of these medications and your physician suspects that your thyroid may be malfunctioning, he or she can easily find out if your active thyroid hormone levels are normal by performing a TSH blood test.

Other Drugs

Interferon and *interleukin* are important new drugs used against certain types of cancer. As described in chapter 3, both drugs play important roles in your body's natural immune defenses as well as in autoimmune disorders. Thus it is not surprising that alterations in thyroid function may be seen in some patients taking these drugs. In one study 21 percent of patients given interleukin-2 and a drug known as *lymphokine-activated killer cells* for advanced cancer became hypothyroid. If one of these drugs is critical for treatment of cancer or another serious medical problem, your doctor can use it but is likely to monitor your thyroid from time to time with examinations and periodic TSH blood tests.

Food

Much has been written about the effect of food upon the thyroid, yet most of what you eat does not present a danger to you. Kelp (which is discussed in the preceding section), may contain large amounts of iodine. Foods of the Brassica family (including cabbage, kale, rutabaga, and turnips) contain a substance that is capable of causing goiter in both animals and humans if their diet is deficient in iodine. Medical research suggests that these foods cause goiter and a decrease in thyroid function because they produce a chemical compound known as *goitrin*, which we know has a negative effect on the thyroid.

Another important foodstuff that may cause goiter in iodine-deficient individuals is the cassava which is a plant commonly eaten in tropical areas. An ingredient of cassava is converted by the body into *thiocyanate*, which can inhibit thyroid function.

These foods may produce goiter in people who live in iodine-deficient areas, but we are not aware of any case in which the thyroid has actually become underactive just because these foods were eaten in an area where there is sufficient dietary iodine.

Some years ago infants who were allergic to milk were given formulas prepared with soy protein instead of milk. Some of these babies developed goiter and thyroid deficiency, but the problem was corrected when extra iodine was added to the formula. Soy formulas are still in use and, with the added iodine, no longer cause thyroid problems in the babies who take them.

STRESS AND EMOTIONS

Physicians have long suspected that stress might play a role in causing the type of hyperthyroidism in which the whole thyroid becomes overactive (diffuse toxic goiter or Graves' disease). Distressing experiences, usually involving a personal loss (such as the death of a loved one or a divorce), often precede the onset of hyperthyroidism and may act as "trigger factors" that precipitate thyroid overactivity in genetically susceptible individuals.

Investigators have found other evidence of a relationship between stress and the thyroid. For example an increase in hyperthyroidism occurred among refugees from Nazi prison camps, as well as among the inhabitants of occupied Denmark during World War II. However, a similar increase in hyperthyroidism was not seen in the Netherlands, which was also occupied by the Nazis, nor has there been an increase in Belfast, Ireland, where there has been a great deal of strife over the last several decades. There have also been experimental studies that have shown changes in thyroid function in animals subjected to stressful conditions, but it is unclear how these studies relate to humans. In spite of all our efforts, however, we still do not know *how* such stress affects the thyroid—just that it seems to "trigger off" thyroid overactivity in some susceptible people.

Physical stresses—such as serious infection, pregnancy, or a surgical operation—may also play a role in the onset of hyperthyroidism in certain individuals. Here, too, although some thyroid specialists accept the idea that such a relationship may exist, we do not know how these physical happenings exert their effect on thyroid function.

There is another side of this too. The hyperthyroidism of Graves' disease can be an extremely stressful emotional experience. As a result the disease can have both immediate and long-term psychiatric consequences for some patients. By the time their thyroid problem is recognized, some individuals have endured months or sometimes years of anxiety, excessive emotional reactions, sleeplessness, weakened muscles, and physical exhaustion. Personal relationships at home or work may have suffered or been permanently altered. A feeling of lack of control over their physical and emotional health may have dominated such patients' lives and seriously damaged their feelings of self-worth.

Patients need time and the support of family, physicians, and friends to recover their emotional stability and begin to trust their bodies again. And it's not easy. Psychiatrists refer to this as a *posttraumatic stress disorder*, and point out that the emotional instability often does not end when the thyroid problem is recognized, or even when blood levels have been restored to normal. A new personal problem or a sleepless night may cause a patient recovering from Graves' disease to wonder whether she is still sick, her condition has worsened, her medication is wrong, or the radioactive iodine or antithyroid drug has permanently changed her. These doubts may revive all of her earlier anxieties as if she were sick all over again.

If you have this problem, don't try to handle it all by yourself. This is an important time to ask others for help. Your physician can measure your thyroid hormone and TSH levels and adjust medication as necessary. Family members must avoid the "here we go again" attitude and help you instead to look for other explanations for your new anxieties or exhaustion. Employers can be helpful with extra time on a project or a day off if you have tried to return to work before you were really healthy. Finally, since much is known about this emotional state, talking with a psychiatrist, a psychologist, or a social worker trained in counseling can be extremely helpful. Therapy of some sort could shorten the time it takes you to regain control of your emotions and begin to trust your feelings about your body again.

SEVERE MEDICAL ILLNESS

If you become seriously ill for more than a week, your physician may well find that your thyroid hormone levels have fallen to much lower levels due to decreased binding of T4 to serum proteins and a decrease in the normal conversion of T4 to T3. Unless you have an underactive thyroid as well, you will maintain adequate blood levels of free or active thyroid hormones, and no treatment is necessary. In that case, although your T4 and T3 levels may decline, your serum TSH will remain normal, confirming a healthy thyroid condition.

ENVIRONMENTAL FACTORS

Much investigation has been carried out to try to understand the effects of such factors as cold, heat, and exercise on the function of your thyroid. This research has shown that none of these environmental factors appears to influence thyroid function to a degree that would significantly affect you even if you had an underlying thyroid problem. Thus your requirement for thyroid hormone does not change in response to a hotter or a colder climate, a change in temperature or altitude, or a change in your physical activity.

OTHER CONSIDERATIONS

A variety of other drugs and environmental factors have been shown to affect the thyroid in some individuals or to change the thyroid function of animals in experimental situations. Fortunately the medical community is very much aware that any new drug must be carefully tested for possible adverse effects of any kind. Indeed such tests, following the guidelines of the Food and Drug Administration, are proving generally effective in preventing thyroid problems in patients taking new drugs. Where problems exist, a treatment is usually available, as is the case when goiter or hypothyroidism develop in patients taking lithium. As a general precaution, however, when you have your periodic health examination, you should be sure to tell your physician about all the drugs, vitamins, and health foods you are taking.

CHAPTER SIXTEEN

Is Your Thyroid Making You Fat?

This chapter is written for you if you are overweight and were told in the past that you were fat because you had an underactive thyroid. Our purpose here is twofold: First, to help you understand why you were told you were hypothyroid in the first place, and second, to help you find out whether you really are hypothyroid now.

When you develop hypothyroidism, you do not, as a rule, also become fat. Your body's use of oxygen (its metabolic rate) decreases, and you may become less physically active than you were when your thyroid was normal; but you probably will not eat enough food to gain a lot of weight. Furthermore, when you are started on thyroid hormone treatment for hypothyroidism, you are not likely to lose much weight, even if you were markedly obese to begin with. There may be a weight loss of three to four pounds early in treatment, but that is due to a loss of accumulated tissue fluid rather than a loss of fat.

Nevertheless you may be taking thyroid hormone tablets today because you, like many other people, were told in the past that you had an underactive thyroid that was causing obesity. Perhaps you will recall having a "breathing test" (basal metabolic rate test, or BMR) or a blood test for protein-bound iodine (PBI), which was interpreted by your physician as being low or in a "borderline range." If you lost weight in the weeks after thyroid hormone treatment was begun, you were probably told that your "clinical trial" on thyroid hormone treatment confirmed the fact that you were indeed hypothyroid.

However, the BMR and PBI tests were not sensitive enough to make a definite diagnosis of hypothyroidism, especially if your thyroid function was only slightly diminished. Obesity itself lowers the BMR and may have given a false impression of hypothyroidism. Physicians now rely on a low blood level of thyroid hormone (thyroxine or T4) and an elevated blood level of the pituitary's thyroid-stimulating hormone to make the diagnosis of mild hypothyroidism. The TSH level, by far the most sensitive indicator of thyroid failure, rises when your pituitary releases TSH into the blood stream because it senses that there is too little thyroid hormone in your blood. Before 1970 it was not possible to measure your serum TSH. Your physician had to rely on less sensitive tests, clinical judgment, and your response to thyroid-hormone treatment. Of course at the time you were first tested, you may have been hypothyroid, and you may still have that problem today. On the other hand you may have always had a normal thyroid gland.

If you lost weight taking thyroid hormone medication, it may have been due to a carefully kept diet rather than to any effect of your thyroid treatment. You may also have experienced a *placebo* effect from your thyroid tablets: *Believing* the tablets would help you lose weight helped you achieve weight loss.

By measuring your serum TSH level now, it is possible to tell with certainty whether you are hypothyroid. This is important to do for three reasons. First, if the diagnosis of hypothyroidism was made by older, less sensitive tests, it is worthwhile to find out if there really is a thyroid problem, for if your thyroid is normal, there is no need to spend money on thyroid medication. Even if you have taken thyroid medication for many years, you can stop it and normal thyroid function will return rapidly if you do not really need it. Second, an excessive dose of thyroid hormone can be a health hazard to you if you are elderly, causing such symptoms as irregular or rapid heartbeat, muscle weakness, nervousness, and difficulty sleeping. Third, if you do have hypothyroidism, you should continue to take thyroid hormone pills for the rest of your life. Your thyroid hormone and TSH blood levels should be measured periodically by your family physician to be sure that your dosage of thyroid hormone is correct. This is important because patients who are mildly hypothyroid when young often experience a greater degree of thyroid deficiency in later life and require a gradual increase in their dosage of thyroid hormone. For these reasons, if you were given thyroid hormone many years ago as treatment for an underactive thyroid or obesity, you should find out now whether your thyroid is normal or not. If it is normal, medication is unnecessary. If it is not normal, your physician can test you and determine what your proper dose of thyroid hormone now should be.

Your physician can easily and safely find out whether you need thyroid treatment by asking you to stop taking your thyroid medication. Six weeks later a sample of your blood can be tested for T4 and TSH. The T4 serves as a general indicator of your thyroid function. It should be low if you are very hypothyroid, but it may be within the "normal range" if your thyroid is only mildly underactive. Your TSH, on the other hand, will *always* be increased above normal if you are hypothyroid, even in a mild degree. Furthermore your serum TSH can be used as a guide to find the correct dose of thyroid hormone for you. Your TSH will be normal if your thyroid is healthy, even if you have taken thyroid hormone tablets for many years.

In summary, if you are a patient who is taking thyroid hormone in the belief that it helps you deal with a weight problem, you are probably wrong. Rather, if you are controlling your weight, the credit is due to you, not the thyroid pills. Nevertheless it is important to find out whether or not your thyroid is normal. By stopping the thyroid treatment and taking a blood test for thyroxine and TSH, under supervision of your physician you will know whether or not you need such medication. If you need thyroid hormone, the dosage should be rechecked periodically. If you don't need it, thyroid tablets represent an unnecessary expense and potential health hazard.

SO IF YOUR THYROID IS OKAY, WHY ARE YOU OVERWEIGHT?

If you are too heavy, it's because you take in more calories than you use up. It has nothing to do with how much anyone else is able to eat and yet stay thin. Rather it depends on your own metabolic state and the factors involved in your personal eating pattern. And as much as scientists want to find one "trigger" that controls food intake, one that they can "turn off" with a drug or treatment, there are many different mechanisms that determine your eating habits. The cure for your weight problem lies in understanding your own particular situation and taking control of it.

How you eat depends first on the way your senses process food: How it looks, smells, and tastes. Then, before you even start to eat, hormonal changes occur in your brain, and secretions of several types of chemicals and hormones take place in your digestive system. These include stomach acid, intestinal enzymes, and insulin from your pancreas, which help digestion and metabolism. Finally, there are feedback systems, which tell us when to stop eating. For some people this may be a "full" feeling as your stomach distends with food. Others may rarely experience much fullness, and only stop eating when nervousness subsides or simply when there is no more food on the table. The long-range feedback systems that tend to keep us at a certain weight are even harder to understand. Some individuals may find little change in their weight even after several weeks or months of eating whatever they feel like, meal after meal.

For a lot of overweight individuals this is not the case. Surveys indicate that 26 percent of adults in the United States, or about thirty-four million people, are overweight. A 1992 National Institutes of Health conference reported that 40 percent of adult women and 24 percent of adult men were trying to lose weight. Since only about 1 percent of them actually weigh less after a year of dieting, it's obviously not easy. So if weight is a problem for you, what can you do to change the odds and slim down?

We think the answer lies in first looking at the factors that seem to be important in your eating pattern. Here a counselor or nutritionist may be helpful. You may not realize how many calories you are taking in with certain foods or alcoholic drinks. Perhaps you're waiting too long to eat and then overeating when you finally have a meal. You may be snacking too much or eating too much fat, which has more than twice the calories of protein or carbohydrates. Sometimes modifications in your behavior patterns may help, such as using a smaller dinner plate, having your spouse serve you, or stopping between-meal snacks.

But perhaps for you it would mean a lot to prove that you *can* lose weight, and that your underlying thyroid problem or another inherited problem has not made you "different from everybody else." To do that, you could try a packaged meal plan, such as Weight Watchers, if your personal physician approves and if you can afford it. If not, ask a nutritionist to suggest a similar program for you to follow with specific meals you make up yourself in exact detail. Just remember that this means you will have to weigh portions, so it will be harder. Set a goal to lose a certain number of pounds. Diet for a fixed time period. We believe that once you find that you really can lose weight, you will have a better chance of success in taking long-term control of your weight problem.

OBESITY

by T. D.

I am presently on my longest and most successful diet to date. However, I've been dieting, with varying degrees of success, for at least ten years. I've fasted, taken diet pills and tranquilizers, drunk ten glasses of water a day, joined Weight Watchers, and eaten grapefruit each meal. I've joined a diet workshop, done the Canadian Air Force exercises, eaten Ayds (I ate a whole box in two days; they tasted great since I wasn't eating much food), joined Weight Watchers again, cut out breakfast, cut out lunch, cut out snacks. I've been offered a new summer wardrobe, a winter, spring, and fall wardrobe. I guess if there was justice in this world, and starting a diet counted for, say, minus five pounds, I'd weigh a hundred pounds today. But I don't (yet). Starting a diet obviously doesn't count. Staying on one does.

Why do I start a diet? I haven't had any of those dramatic, impressive, catastrophic reasons that we've all heard of. I've never been unable to buckle an airline seat belt, or had a heart attack, or been caught in a revolving door, or been unable to find anything to fit me while shopping. There's always the Chubby Shop. For me it's usually been an accumulation of things: Never looking as good or as well tailored as my roommate. (Why do fat people always have thin roommates?) Standing pretty much alone at a college mixer, trying to pretend I really prefer listening to the music. Having a solicitous saleslady suggest that something a little fuller might be more flattering to my figure (or lack thereof) Having my mother tell me that the dress I finally, finally bought looks positively matronly. Periodically these things all run together; I get depressed and upset enough about my excess fat to try to do something about it.

So, I'd start another diet. (I don't object at all to the word *diet*. Call it an *eating program*, a *balanced nutritional pattern*, or whatever; it's a diet. Why play with words?) Any diet is pretty easy for the first few days. I'm generally carried along on a wave of self-satisfaction, encouragement from others, and the pleasure of discovering that I do, after all, have willpower and *can* lose weight. I think most people who want to lose weight know pretty much how they should eat. A good breakfast, sugar substitute in the coffee, one slice of toast, easy on the margarine. A salad, maybe some meat and fruit for lunch. Meat, fish, poultry, vegetables for dinner. No snacks, no desserts, and so on. We've been taught it in school, heard it on TV, read it in the popular magazines. But for me, again and again, while I know all this, it still hasn't worked.

But it is possible to lose weight successfully and not gain it back. If you're aware of the danger signals, you can take steps to counteract them:

1. Don't start on a diet without thinking it through. Go to a doctor on the chance that there might be a medical reason for your fat. Don't start on an impulse, because the momentum will not last long.

2. Pick a sensible diet and plan on something you can stay with for a long time. Could you really eat grapefruit for the rest of your life?

3. Be patient and try to take a long-range view. Aim for, say, five pounds in a month, one hundred pounds in two years. This, I think, is the hardest part, but it's the only rational approach to take.

4. Have someone to talk to. Not your friends or coworkers, since they're interested, but generally pretty bored by endless talk of dieting. Go to a group meeting, or a doctor, or talk to people who've lost a lot of weight themselves. I've found them to be pretty sympathetic and encouraging listeners. Note: I've found that it's disastrous to go food shopping when you're at a low point, morale-wise. Everything looks so good! And then you feel obligated to eat all that junk you bought so that you don't waste the money you spent.

5. Find other ways to cheer yourself up. This is generally more time-consuming and requires more thought than just going to the refrigerator. Whatever you pick (a walk, a bike ride, a museum, a tennis game, shopping) usually has the added benefit of involving at least minimal physical exertion.

6. If none of the above works and you're really fed up (I think this is almost inevitable in any long diet), go ahead and indulge, but set a ceiling of five to ten pounds gained before you start again in earnest. In the overall picture this is lost time, but sometimes it is the only way. I know that after a few days of indulging myself after months of dieting, I usually feel guilty and annoyed at myself and start back in again.

In summary I find my two main problems in dieting are these:

1. Impatience.

2. Feeling guilty and depressed. After about six months of consistent progress the impatience pretty much goes away. The guilty feelings stay around as long as I go off and on any diet. I used to think I had absolutely no will-power, no motivation, and couldn't finish something I'd started. That's a pretty depressing opinion to have of yourself. But with long experience I've realized that diet-ing is *hard*. Worth it, but hard. Slipping occasionally is permissible, as long as it's not too often nor too far.

If dieting were easy, no one would be fat.

CHAPTER SEVENTEEN

Future Research Directions

Researchers have made enormous advances in learning
about the thyroid over the last thirty years, but we still have
a long way to go in understanding how thyroid hormones
work and why the thyroid is so susceptible to malfunction.
In this final chapter we will briefly review current research
in the thyroid field.

THYROID-HORMONE ACTION

When we talk about thyroid hormone action, we mean the
manner in which the thyroid hormones exert their effect on
the body. At the present time we believe that these hormones exert most of their effects by going directly to the
nucleus of cells. Within the nucleus the hormones bind to
very specific receptors. Some tissues have many thyroid
hormone receptors while others have few or none. The degree to which a tissue responds to thyroid hormone is at
least partially determined by how many receptors are present in the cells. For example, the heart has a large number
of thyroid-hormone receptors and is very sensitive to thyroid hormone; the spleen and gonads do not have many receptors and are relatively insensitive to changes in thyroidal
status.

But how does the interaction between thyroid hormones
with their nuclear receptors change the function of an or-
gan? This is a very important question and one that researchers are trying very hard to answer. Currently most
investigators believe that the thyroid-hormone/receptor
complex goes to specific genes, which are pieces of our genetic material (DNA) that encode proteins in a given tissue,

and turns the gene on or off. Thus thyroid hormones could directly affect how a given tissue functions by altering gene activity within that tissue. Exactly how this occurs at a molecular level is not yet fully understood, but consider how important this discovery might be! If we understood how to control genes, we might then be able to selectively activate a certain set of genes to combat certain illnesses. For example heart failure is a deadly health problem without a known cure. Suppose we could turn on the genes in the heart that caused the heart muscle to grow or to contract more strongly. That would be a monumental achievement of great benefit to humankind.

AUTOIMMUNITY—
WHY THE THYROID GETS SICK

We know many facts about the symptoms of thyroid diseases but far too little about what causes them. For example women get hyperthyroidism and hypothyroidism four to eight times as often as men. Why? To be honest, we do not have a clue. These same thyroid diseases tend to run in families, suggesting a genetic factor. In fact, most researchers believe that genetics are the most important factor in causing thyroid disease. As we reviewed earlier, autoimmunity occurs when the body turns its immune system against its own natural tissues, such as the thyroid gland. This results in T cells and antibodies directed against thyroid cells. Why does this occur? Some researchers believe that a mutation (a small change in a gene) occurs in a gene that is important for thyroid function. This mutated gene then yields a thyroid protein that is slightly changed by the mutation and is perceived by the body's immune surveillance system as a foreign or altered protein (see Chapter 3). When the body's immune system sees this abnormality in protein structure, it views the mutation as a foreign substance and initiates an immune reaction to it. T cells and antibodies against the thyroid are thus formed that attack the thyroid and either cause the gland to malfunction or else destroy it.

So what do researchers do? They look very carefully for

changes or mutations in proteins that are important for the thyroid. They do this by first isolating the genes that encode these proteins and then looking for mutations. Imagine the potential for this approach. If a mutation is found, one very important direct benefit would be the ability to tell whether the same mutation is present in other family members. For example, when a mutation is discovered that can be linked to hyperthyroidism or hypothyroidism, whole families could be screened. Babies could be tested at birth to tell who is at risk and who is safe. The next step would be to introduce a correction of the mutation, which might then prevent the disease from ever occurring. It sounds like magic, but it is just beyond the horizon if biomedical genetic research is adequately funded.

THYROID TUMORS

As noted earlier, thyroid tumors (mostly benign) occur in 50 percent of the population, and the chance of having one grow to the point of being clinically important is one in ten. We don't know why these tumors are so common. One theory is that the thyroid gland itself produces substances that cause nodules to grow in an autonomous fashion, beyond the control of TSH. What are these substances? Some researchers call them *oncogenes*, or tumor-promoting factors. There is a very important body of research that suggests that these factors may be very important in thyroid tumor development. The trick is to find the oncogenes and learn how to control their expression. To date we have found no definitive answer and thus no solution to the prevention of thyroid nodules or thyroid cancer. But there are hints. New oncogenes have recently been found that are associated with papillary and medullary thyroid cancers. Furthermore even benign "hot nodules" have sometimes been found to be associated with changes in growth-promoting factors. Thus in the next few years biomedical research may uncover some of the mysteries surrounding thyroid cancer development, and therefore affect its prevention or cure.

THYROID HORMONE AND THE BRAIN

The brain is one of the most important targets for thyroid-hormone action. The thyroid influences the ability to think, calculate, and develop emotional reactions. Also certain psychiatric diseases are related to thyroid gland malfunction. Research in this area is in an embryonic stage at present. We do not have a clear idea of exactly what functions in the brain are controlled by thyroid hormones. More important we have not yet identified which brain-specific proteins to study, so we really do not know what genes would be most informative. But again, use your imagination; consider the potential in being able to control or stimulate genes that are directly linked to concentration, memory functions, or depression. We predict that in the next decade doctors will make enormous new advances in our understanding of how thyroid hormone affects the brain, and these discoveries will lead the way toward new therapies for depression and other cognitive disorders.

THYROID CANCER

A very direct benefit is right around the corner for patients with thyroid cancer. Until now you have had to stop thyroid medicine for two to six weeks before you have a radioiodine scan to look for cancer recurrence. This often makes you feel relatively tired and sluggish due to hypothyroidism. Genetic engineering has developed a new human TSH molecule that will allow physicians to perform scans to test for recurrence without discontinuing your thyroid medicine for even one day. This new genetically engineered molecule is very close to being approved for use in patients with thyroid cancer, thus greatly simplifying the test for cancer recurrence.

These are just a few of the new directions in thyroid research that are being explored today. We look forward to being able to share more exciting discoveries with you in the very near future as we learn more about how the thyroid affects our bodies and how diseases of the thyroid are triggered.

APPENDIX ONE

Choosing a Thyroid Surgeon

Your physician may refer you to a surgeon for help with a number of thyroid problems. You may have an overactive thyroid that has not responded to medical treatment, and there may be reasons for not taking treatment with radioactive iodine. You may have a very large thyroid, or goiter, that is disfiguring or interfering with breathing or swallowing. You may have a nodule or lump in your thyroid, and your physician wants a biopsy to tell if it contains cancer. You may have a thyroid tumor that needs to be removed, or a recurrence of a previous cancer.

Several types of surgeons operate on the thyroid, including general surgeons, otolaryngologists (ear, nose, and throat specialists), cancer surgeons, thoracic (chest) surgeons, and even surgeons who specialize in operating on patients with endocrine problems. On the other hand your problem could be Graves' disease and you may need eye surgery. Here an ophthalmologist or plastic surgeon may be the best choice. Any one of these could be right for your problem.

The most important considerations for you and your physician are the type and extent of your problem and the skill and experience a particular surgeon offers. Here are some questions to ask: Has the surgeon had good results with your type of problem? Does the doctor have special training in endocrine operations or neck surgery? How often does he or she do this type of operation? Does the surgeon have special credentials, such as board certification or membership in the American Association of Endocrine Surgeons? What is the surgeon's complication rate for problems such as injury to the laryngeal nerve, which supplies the vocal cords, or to the parathyroid glands?

There is another way of looking at this too. In this era of "managed" health care, insurance companies are taking an increasingly active role in deciding who should perform surgery of many types. But in your special circumstance of thyroid surgery, which can be unexpectedly delicate and complicated, not everyone who does thyroid operations will be right for you. Make sure that the choice of the surgeon is matched to the operation that is to be performed.

To give you a place to begin discussions with your physician and, if necessary, your insurance company, you might consider the following guidelines:

- A general surgeon who does less than ten thyroid operations per year could do a thyroid biopsy or remove small cysts and benign (noncancerous) tumors confined to one thyroid lobe.

- A surgeon who does at least ten to fifteen thyroid operations per year could be right for benign goiter, thyroid cancer consisting of a single nodule less than an inch in diameter confined to one thyroid lobe, or a near-total thyroidectomy for uncomplicated hyperthyroidism.

- Only a surgeon who has performed more than one hundred thyroid operations (excluding biopsy) should be chosen for a large obstructive goiter under your breastbone (substernal goiter), reoperation for recurrent cancer, thyroid cancers larger than an inch in diameter (these are more likely to have spread locally), any medullary thyroid cancer, or anaplastic (rapidly spreading) cancer.

Remember, these are only guidelines. A particularly gifted surgeon in your area may be right for your problem, even though he or she does not fit into an exact category. In that case ask your physician to explain the reasons for choosing that surgeon for you. These ideas are presented to help you understand your particular surgical needs and to provide a starting point for discussion with your physician about your surgeon.

Above all, your physician is in the best position to help you with this important decision.

APPENDIX TWO

Guidelines for Patients Receiving Radioiodine Therapy

If your physician has recommended that you be treated with radioactive iodine for an overactive thyroid or for a thyroid tumor, you will be given a larger dose of radioactive material than the tiny amounts used for thyroid testing. Therefore you will want to discuss any needed precautions with your physician, depending on your particular situation, diagnosis, and the dose of radioactive iodine planned for you.

There are some general guidelines, however, that you could use as the basis for discussion and planning before you are treated. They are based on the fact that the iodine will remain in your thyroid in your neck for a few days and will leave your body mainly in your urine. It can also be found in your blood, saliva, and breast milk, and can cross the placenta to an unborn baby if you are pregnant.

During the first three days after treatment:

- Drink at least four glasses of water or other liquids each day.

- Wash your hands carefully before preparing food for other people.

- Use separate bath linens to avoid contamination of others.

- Any disposable paper products that may have been contaminated with saliva, blood, urine, or mucus (such as sanitary napkins) should be flushed down the toilet or discarded in a plastic bag.

207

- Wash your hands after going to the toilet and then rinse the sink with water.

- Try to stay two to three feet away from other people.

- If you are breast-feeding, stop. Ask your doctor when you may resume (usually in about one or two months). Ask your obstetrician about ways to avoid breast discomfort.

- Sleep alone if possible. Avoid kissing and sexual relations.

- If you care for a baby, limit your contact to less than two hours a day.

- Dispose of all tissues down the toilet immediately after use.

- Avoid pregnancy for about six months. Ask your doctor about this, for there may be special circumstances to consider in planning pregnancy relating to your particular thyroid problem.

APPENDIX THREE

The Cost of Thyroid Testing

The cost of thyroid tests and procedures varies considerably among hospitals and independent laboratories and should be a consideration in thyroid diagnosis and treatment not only of health insurers and hospitals but also of physicians and patients as well. In the following comments references to the cost of testing are based on a random survey of several hospitals rather than an exhaustive study of the economics of testing and procedures throughout the United States comparing physicians' offices, independent laboratories, and small and large hospitals. Our purpose is to indicate the importance of cost as a factor in thyroid diagnosis and treatment. We urge the patients and health professionals who read these words to adapt our suggestions and comments to the expense profiles within their own health care system.

THYROID SCREENING

There are certain occasions when large numbers of patients are screened for evidence of thyroid dysfunction. Surveying for thyroid dysfunction is common among elderly individuals, among women over fifty, and among women who have just had a baby. If a TSH test is the only test used to look for thyroid dysfunction, it will probably cost about $50 (range $43 to $89 in our survey). If a physician measures additional hormone levels, the cost will be higher: T_4—$17 to $29, T_3—$43 to $91, and free T_4—$36 to $41. Thus the latter tests should be done only if the TSH is low, suggesting hyperthyroidism, or high, suggesting hypothyroidism. These other hormone values would generally be used to evaluate the severity of the disease only if the TSH confirms that the thyroid is malfunctioning.

SCANS AND X RAYS

In our survey a radioiodine (^{123}I) uptake and scan cost between $354 and $417; a technetium uptake and scan $162 to $446; a thyroid ultrasound $152 to $454; a CT scan $267 to $588; and an MRI $796 to $1,357. Thus your physician may choose one or another of these procedures depending on their cost in your area. The figures above should help you realize why thyroid ultrasound is an increasingly common way to follow patients with thyroid cancer and is often preferred to the more expensive alternative procedures.

THYROID BIOPSY

The cost of a thyroid biopsy in most hospitals is about $500, but may vary dramatically among institutions and also within one hospital, since it depends not only on the professional charge from the physician performing the biopsy but also on highly variable charges from the cytology department. Biopsy costs will increase according to the number of samples taken and any need for special tissue stains on the samples obtained. Yet a biopsy is quite a cost-effective procedure if the tissue obtained is found to be harmless (benign), saving you from having a thyroid operation.

THYROID SURGERY

The cost of thyroid surgery depends mostly on the number of days you are in the hospital and the number of hours you are in the operating room. Thus a lobectomy (two-hour operation and two days in the hospital) in our survey costs between $4,100 and $8,000. In contrast a total thyroidectomy requiring four hours in the operating room and a three-day hospital stay, costs from $5,350 to $18,000 in the hospitals we surveyed. You can see that if removal of a single thyroid lobe and its nodule is adequate treatment for a papillary cancer, there are financial constraints that should compel surgeons to limit themselves to that procedure rather than performing the longer and more complex total thyroidectomy in such patients. If radioactive-iodine treatment or whole-body scanning is necessary, remaining thyroid tissue in the neck can usually be destroyed by radioiodine treatment at lower cost as effectively, and sometimes more safely, than a surgeon performing total thyroidectomy.

RADIOIODINE TREATMENT

The cost of radioiodine (^{131}I) treatment for hyperthyroidism ranged in our survey from $417 to $560, considerably less than the cost of a thyroid operation to cure this condition. But if your problem is thyroid cancer, your physician may need to give you larger doses of radioiodine. In that case hospitalization may be required until most of the radioactivity has left your body and you no longer represent a radioactive risk to those around you. In such a case the total cost including hospitalization and the precautions required to handle the radioactive materials ranged from $1,061 to $3,592.

USE OF "OUTSIDE" LABORATORIES FOR SCREENING

A "best buy" in thyroid screening could be the test for antimicrosomal (antiperoxidase) thyroid antibodies in pregnant women. The cost of the test in our survey ranged from $22 to $99. At $22 it would make a good screening test in pregnant women. If the test is positive, their risk for postpartum thyroid dysfunction increases from 5 to 45 percent, and careful follow-up with TSH testing after delivery would be essential. If your doctor works at a hospital where the cost of the test is $99, one might make a case for sending your blood sample to an outside laboratory where the test could be done at a more reasonable rate.

Financial considerations such as these will become increasingly important in years to come as all of us try to deliver good medical care at a reasonable cost. We hope that these comments give you some perspective of the ways doctors and patients can approach the financial aspects of medical care together.

APPENDIX FOUR

The Thyroid Foundation of America, Inc.

If you have found this volume helpful, we hope you will consider membership in the Thyroid Foundation of America as a way of continuing your education and expanding your understanding about your thyroid condition. Most thyroid problems are lifelong and tend to change over time. New information from thyroid research may lead to recommendations to change treatment for certain conditions. Furthermore there are many related autoimmune conditions (such as diabetes, pernicious anemia, and vitiligo) about which many thyroid patients ought to keep up-to-date.

The Thyroid Foundation of America was created in 1985 to

- Provide health education and support to thyroid patients and the health professionals who care for them

- Increase public awareness about thyroid problems

- Raise and distribute funds to find the causes, cures, and ultimately the means of preventing thyroid disorders

Membership benefits in the Thyroid Foundation of America include

- Periodic newsletters with up-to-date articles about important thyroid topics, information on new thyroid research, reviews of new thyroid books for patients, and an "Ask the Doctor" column, in which patients' questions are answered

- Occasional bulletins with updated information on specific conditions

- Referrals to endocrinologists in your geographic area

- Assistance in forming support groups, Thyroid Interest Groups, and TFA Chapters in your area

- Information on thyroid books and publications

Membership will run for one year from receipt of your membership application.

Regular Member $25
Student..$15
Senior Citizen..$15
Physician..$75
Other Health Professional $25

Your dues and any tax-deductible donation you make to TFA enables the foundation to continue your education, supports TFA's outreach programs in public and patient education, and enables TFA to be there for anyone with a thyroid problem.

Be sure to enclose your name, address, and telephone number. By mentioning your thyroid diagnosis and other areas of interest in thyroidology, you will be enrolled in programs that also provide you occasional bulletins about new information concerning your condition. As a special bonus new members receive their choice among three books about the thyroid written for patients, so write to TFA and join today.

The Thyroid Foundation of America, Inc.
Ruth Sleeper Hall RSL 350 Box YT
40 Parkman Street
Boston MA 02114-2698

Phone: 617-726-8500
        800-832-8321
Fax: 617-726-4136

APPENDIX FIVE

Thyroid Statistics

(Prepared by the Thyroid Foundation of America, Inc.)*
(Reprinted with permission of The Thyroid Foundation of America, Inc.)

THYROID DYSFUNCTION

Twenty to 25 percent of the population in the United States has a tendency toward autoimmune disorders. Many of these people develop hyperthyroidism or hypothyroidism. Among these people the first signs of thyroid failure is an increase in the blood level of thyroid-stimulating hormone (TSH).

HYPERTHYROIDISM: GRAVES' DISEASE

This condition is five times more common in women than in men.

Women (over age fifteen)

Prevalence—Recognized and treated	3.2%	(3,221,760)
—Unrecognized	0.5%	(503,000)
Annual Incidence (new cases/ year)	0.3%	(302,040)

Men (over age fifteen)

Prevalence—Recognized and treated	0.32%	(289,000)
—Unrecognized	0.05%	(46,320)
Annual Incidence (new cases/ year)	0.03%	(27,852)

*According to 1990 census data.

HYPOTHYROIDISM
(Severe illness requiring treatment)
This condition is five times more common in women than in men.

Women (over age fifteen)

Prevalence—Recognized and treated	1.47%	(1,409,502)
—Unrecognized	0.33%	(332,244)
Annual Incidence (new cases/year)	0.15%	(151,020)

Men (over age fifteen)

Prevalence—Recognized and treated	0.1%	(92,840)
—Unrecognized	0.033%	(30,637)
Annual Incidence (new cases/year)	0.015%	(13,926)

SUBCLINICAL HYPOTHYROIDISM
This condition is five times more common in women than in men, and usually recognized because it produces so few symptoms.

By age fifty, 10 percent of women have an increased blood level of TSH, a sensitive sign that the thyroid may be failing.	5,910,700	women
By age sixty as many as 16.9 percent of women and 8.7 percent of men have an increased blood level of TSH.	2,000,000	women
	1,479,000	men

OVERALL PREVALENCE OF RECOGNIZED THYROID DISEASE

Women and men	5,013,120

OVERALL PREVALENCE OF UNRECOGNIZED THYROID DISEASE

Women and men

Severe illness	912,200
Subclinical hypothyroidism	6,839,000
TOTAL	7,851,000

Thus 13 million Americans have an overactive or underactive thyroid and more than half, or nearly 8 million of them, do not realize they are sick.

POSTPARTUM THYROIDITIS

The thyroid commonly malfunctions after pregnancy. A woman has a 5 percent chance of becoming either hyper- or hypothyroid after delivery, and this may be a cause of postpartum depression. Since there are approximately 4,000,000 women in the United States who become pregnant each year, this means that 200,000 of them develop thyroid dysfunction after delivery. The incidence of this condition increases to 25 percent if the woman has evidence of another autoimmune disorder, such as insulin-dependent diabetes mellitus.

It is therefore especially important to follow women carefully during the postpartum period if they or family members have insulin-dependent diabetes, rheumatoid arthritis, pernicious anemia, prematurely gray hair, vitiligo, and so on. Many physicians obtain a blood sample early in pregnancy to test for the presence of antithyroid antibodies. If antibodies are found, the likelihood of postpartum thyroid dysfunction is increased. Careful follow-up after delivery is indicated.

IODINE DEFICIENCY AND GOITER

One billion people (one-fifth of the world's population) live in areas where they are at risk for dietary iodine deficiency that could lead to goiter, mental deficiency, decreased academic performance for children, and decreased economic productivity in their community. Although iodine deficiency is unknown in the United States due to our iodine-rich diets, at least 200 million people worldwide have goiter, most of which is due to iodine deficiency.

NODULES

Thyroid lumps are common. Fifty percent of the population will have a nodule sometime during their lifetime, although most of these are never detected. Four percent have a nodule now that could be detected in a careful neck examination. Most are harmless. Some can produce thyroid hormone and cause hyperthyroidism. Some are cancerous. Both conditions require treatment.

THYROID CANCER

- Twenty-five people per million develop new thyroid cancers each year (six thousand cases)
- 0.6% of all cancer in men
- 1.6% of all cancer in women

CHILDHOOD NECK IRRADIATION

Two million people in the United States had X-ray treatments to the head or neck area for such conditions as acne, thymus enlargement, recurrent tonsillitis, and chronic ear infections. They are now at risk for thyroid nodules and thyroid cancer. Individuals are especially at risk if they become hypothyroid, for in that situation increased production of TSH from the pituitary gland may stimulate the development and growth of thyroid nodules and cancers.

NEONATAL HYPOTHYROIDISM

About one in every four thousand babies is born with hypothyroidism. Almost all of these newborns are identified shortly after birth through an effective national screening program by means of a thyroid blood test. If hypothyroid newborns are treated with thyroid hormone within two months, complications of mental deficiency, poor growth, and abnormal development usually can be prevented. These children need to continue thyroid treatment and follow-up examinations lifelong.

If you have questions about the above information, please write to the Thyroid Foundation of America. Send a

*stamped self-addressed business-sized envelope with your
inquiry. (The address of TFA is on page 213.)*

The statistics in this article were drawn from the 1990 report of the U.S. Bureau of the Census and the following
references:

Articles from *The Bridge*, a quarterly publication of the
Thyroid Foundation of America, Inc., Boston, Massachusetts.

Braverman, Lewis E., and Robert D. Utiger. Werner and
Ingbar's *The Thyroid, A Fundamental and Clinical Text*,
6th ed. (Philadelphia: J. B. Lippincott Company, 1991).

Tunbridge, Michael G., et al., "The Spectrum of Thyroid
Disease in a Community: The Whickham Survey," *Clinical Endocrinology* 7 (1977): 481.

Wood, Lawrence C., David S. Cooper, and E. Chester
Ridway. *Your Thyroid, A Home Reference*, (New York:
Ballantine Books, 1995).

APPENDIX SIX

Suggested Reading About Thyroid Disorders

BOOKS FOR PATIENTS AND THE GENERAL PUBLIC

Baskin, H. Jack. *How Your Thyroid Works*, 3rd ed. Chicago: Adams Press, 1991.

Bayliss, R.I.S., and W.M.G. Tunbridge. *Thyroid Disease: The Facts*, 2nd ed. New York: Oxford University Press, 1991.

Hamburger, Joel I. *The Thyroid Gland: A Book for Thyroid Patients*, 7th ed. Published privately by Dr. Hamburger, 1991.

Surks, Martin I. *The Thyroid Book: What Goes Wrong and How to Treat It*. Yonkers, N.Y.: Consumer Reports Books, 1994.

MEDICAL TEXTBOOKS ABOUT THE THYROID

Braverman, Lewis E., and Robert D. Utiger, eds. *Werner and Inbar's The Thyroid: A Fundamental and Clinical Text*, 6th ed. Philadelphia: J. B. Lippincott Company, 1991.

Burrow, Gerard W., Jack H. Oppenheimer, and Robert Volpé. *Thyroid Function and Disease*. Philadelphia: W. B. Saunders Company, 1989.

DeGroot, Leslie J., and John B. Stanbury. *The Thyroid and Its Diseases*, 5th ed. New York: John Wiley & Sons, Inc., 1984.

Green, William L., ed. *The Thyroid*. New York: Elsevier Science Publishing Company, Inc., 1986.

Hamburger, Joel I. *Management of Thyroid Patients*, 2nd ed. 2 vols. Published privately by Dr. Hamburger, 1985.

General Endocrinology and Special Topics

Cady, Blake, and Ricardo L. Rossi. *Surgery of the Thyroid and Parathyroid Glands*, 3rd ed. Philadelphia: W. B. Saunders Company, 1991.

Clark, Orlo H. *Endocrine Surgery of the Thyroid and Parathyroid Glands*. St. Louis: C. V. Mosby Company, 1985.

DeGroot, Leslie J. ed. *Endocrinology*, 3rd ed. Philadelphia: W. B. Saunders Company, 1994.

Felig, Phillip, John D. Baxter, and Lawrence A. Frohman. *Endocrinology and Metabolism*. New York: McGraw-Hill Inc., 1994.

Gorman, Colum A., Robert R. Waller, and John A. Dyer, eds. *The Eye and Orbit in Thyroid Disease*. New York: Raven Press, 1984.

Greenspan, Francis, and John Baxter, eds. *Basic and Clinical Endocrinology*, 4th ed. Norwalk, Conn.: Appleton and Lange, 1994.

Kaplan, Solomon A. *Clinical Pediatric Endocrinology*. Philadelphia: W. B. Saunders Company, 1990.

Volpé, Robert. "Immunology of Human Thyroid Disease." In Volpé, R., ed. *Autoimmunity in Endocrine Diseases*. Boca Raton: CRC Press, 1990.

Wilson, Jean D., and Daniel W. Foster. *Williams' Textbook of Endocrinology*, 8th ed. Philadelphia: W. B. Saunders Company, 1992.

APPENDIX SEVEN

Important Organizations You Should Know About

THYROID ORGANIZATIONS FOR PATIENTS

Thyroid Foundation of America
Ruth Sleeper Hall RSL 350
40 Parkman Street
Boston, MA 02114-2698
Phone: 617-726-8500; 800-832-8321
Fax: 617-726-4136

National Graves' Disease Foundation
2 Tsitsi Court
Brevard, NC 28712
(Contact Executive Director Nancy Patterson, Ph.D., for information about support groups for patients who have Graves' disease but note that the NGDF may merge with TFA in 1995, so call or write TFA if you cannot locate the NGDF.)

The Thyroid Society
7515 South Main Street, Suite 545
Houston, TX 77030
Phone: 713-799-9909

CHAPS (Congenital Hypothyroidism And Parent Support)
Sheila Ann Martin, Founder
8 Rock Hill Court
Edwardsville, IL 62025

INTERNATIONAL ORGANIZATIONS FOR PATIENTS
Thyroid Foundation of Canada
1040 Gardiners Road, Suite C
Kingston, Ontario
K7P1R7 Canada
Phone: 613-634-3426
Fax: 613-634-3483

The British Thyroid Foundation
P.O. Box HP22
Leeds
LS6 3RT England

Thyroid Eye Disease (TED)
Lea House
21 Troarn Way
Chudleigh, Chaidleigh-town, Devon-county Devon
TQ13 OPP England
Phone: 0626-852-980

Forum Schilddrüse e. V.
Prof. Dr. med. P. Pfannenstiel
Anna-Birle-Strasse 1 (Am Petersweg)
D-55252 Wiesbaden/Mainz-Kastel
Germany

Schildklierstichting Nederland
Postbus 138
1620 AC Hoom
Nederlands

**ORGANIZATIONS FOR PHYSICIANS AND
HEALTH PROFESSIONALS**
American Thyroid Association, Inc.
Montefiore Medical Center
111 East 210th Street
Bronx, NY 10467
Phone: 718-882-6047
Fax: 718-882-6085

American Association of Clinical Endocrinologists
2589 Park Street
Jacksonville, FL 32204-4554
Phone: 904-384-9490
Fax: 904-384-8124

The Endocrine Society
4350 East West Highway
Suite 500
Bethesda, MD 20814-4410
Phone: 301-941-0200
Fax: 301-941-0259

Endocrine Nurses' Society
P.O. Box 229
West Linn, OR 97068
Phone: 503-494-3714

OTHER ORGANIZATIONS TO KNOW ABOUT

Addison News
(Newsletter for Addison patients)
6142 Territorial Road
Pleasant Lake, MI 49272

American Autoimmune Related Diseases Assoc., Inc.
Michigan National Bank Bldg.
15475 Gratiot Ave.
Detroit, MI 48205
Phone: 313-371-8600
Fax: 313-372-1512

American Cancer Society
1599 Clifton Road
N.E. Atlanta, GA 30329
Phone: 800-ACS-2345

American Heart Association
7272 Greenville Avenue
Dallas, TX 75231
Phone: 214-373-6300

Arthritis Foundation
1314 Spring Street, N.W.
Atlanta, GA 30309
Phone: 800-283-7800

Asthma and Allergy Foundation of America
1125 15th Street, N.W., Suite 502
Washington, DC 20005
Phone: 800-7-ASTHMA
       202-466-7643

Carpal Tunnel Association
4301 Garden City Drive, Suite 301
Landover, MD 20785
Phone: 800-964-8088
Fax: 301-731-0652

Cancer Information Service
Office of Cancer Communication
NCI/NIH
Building 31 10A24
900 Rockville Place
Bethesda, MD 20892
Phone: 1-800-4-CANCER

American Diabetes Association
1660 Duke Street
Alexandria, VA 22314
Phone: 800-232-3472, ext. 366-341

Juvenile Diabetes Foundation, International
432 Park Avenue South
New York, NY 10016
Phone: 212-889-7575

Crohn's and Colitis Foundation
386 Park Avenue South, 17th Floor
New York, NY 10016
Phone: 800-932-2423

International Council for Control of Iodine Deficiency
    Disorders (ICCIDD)
Newsletter and Information:
J.T. Dunn, M.D.
Box 511, University of Virginia Medical Center
Charlottesville, VA 22908

Lupus Foundation of America
4 Research Place, Suite 180
Rockville, MD 20850
Phone: 800-558-0121
Information line: 301-670-9292

Magic Foundation
1327 North Harlem Avenue
Oak Park, IL 60302
Phone: 800-3-MAGIC-3
*(National nonprofit for parents, whose children have
    medical conditions affecting their growth)*

Multiple Sclerosis Foundation
601 Whitehorse Pike
Oaklyn, NJ 08107
Phone: 800-833-4672

National Adrenal Diseases Foundation
505 Northern Boulevard
Great Neck, NY 11021
Phone: 586-487-4992

National Mental Health Association
1021 Prince Street
Alexandria, VA 22314-2971
Phone: 800-969-6642
Fax: 703-684-5968

National Organization for Rare Disorders
P.O. Box 8923
New Fairfield, CT 06812-1783
Phone: 800-999-NORD
203-746-6518
203-746-6481

National Sjögren's Syndrome Foundation, Inc.
3333 N. Broadway
Jericho, NY 11753
Phone: 516-933-6365

Sjögren's Syndrome Foundation
3201 West Evans Dr.
Phoenix, AZ 85023
Phone: 602-516-0787

National Vitiligo Foundation
P.O. Box 6337
Tyler, TX 75711
Phone: 903-534-2925
Fax: 903-534-8075

Pituitary Tumor Network Association
38 S. Wendy Drive
Newbury Park, CA 91320
Phone: 805-499-9973

Scleroderma Federation
Peabody Office Building
1 Newbury Street
Peabody, MA 01960
Phone: 508-535-6600

APPENDIX EIGHT

Some Useful Information

ABBREVIATIONS

T_3—**Triiodothyronine** Thyroid hormones

T_4—**Thyroxine**

T_3 **Suppression Test**—A thyroid test in which a patient takes T_3 tablets in an attempt to reduce thyroid function

THBI—Thyroid-hormone binding index & T_3 Resin Uptake—Both of these tests evaluate the degree to which thyroid hormones are bound to blood proteins

Free T4 Index (T7)—A mathematical calculation derived by multiplying the $T_4 \times T_3$ resin uptake that is done in order to evaluate thyroid function

TSH—Thyroid stimulating hormone

TRH—TSH releasing hormone, used for testing pituitary-thyroid relationship

RAI—radioactive iodine, used for testing and treating the thyroid

RAIU—radioactive iodine uptake, a thyroid function test

^{131}**I**, ^{123}**I**—Radioactive isotopes of iodine

^{99m}**Tc**—radioactive technetium, a radioactive isotope sometimes used in place of radioiodine in the performance of thyroid scans

NORMAL LABORATORY VALUES

Normal values vary considerably from laboratory to laboratory, and therefore tests can only be interpreted if the normal ranges for the laboratory where they were performed are known. A given range of normal (e.g., T4: 4.7–11.1 µg/dl) means that 95 percent of a normal population of people will have T4 values within those limits. The normal ranges for common thyroid blood tests at the Massachusetts General Hospital Thyroid Unit are as follows:

T4: 4.7–11.1µg/dl
T3: 75–195 ng/dl
THBI: 0.77–1.23
T3 resin uptake: 25%–35%
Free T4 Index: 1–4
Free T4: 0.8–1.9 ng/dl
TSH: 0.5–5.0 mU/mi
Radioiodine ^{123}I uptake: 10–30%/24 hr.
Thyroid antiperoxide (antimicrosomal) antibody: 0

DRUGS USED BY THYROID PATIENTS

Thyroid Hormones
Thyroxine (T4)—Levoxyl, Levothroid, Synthroid, Eltroxin
Triiodothyronine (T3)—Cytomel
Desiccated thyroid—powdered animal thyroid
T3–T4 mixture—Thyrolar

Antithyroid Drugs
Propylthiouracil—often just referred to as PTU
Methimazole—Tapazole
Carbimazole—similar to Tapazole and used in England and Europe

Beta-Adrenergic-Blocking Drugs That Block the Action of Thyroid Hormones in Body Tissues
Short-acting:
Propranolol—Inderal
Long-acting:
Acebutalol—Sectral
Atenolol—Tenormin
Metaprolol— Lopressor
Nadolol—Corgard
Propranalol (long-acting)—Inderal-LA
Timolol—Blocadren

Iodine Preparations
Potassium iodide
Saturated solution of potassium iodide—may be referred
to also as SSKI
Lugol's solution

Some Other Important Drugs Mentioned in This Book
Amiodarone—a heart drug that contains iodine and thus
may affect thyroid function
Lithium—an antidepressant drug that may affect thyroid
function
Psoralens—used to treat vitiligo
Vitamin B12—used to treat pernicious anemia
(combined-systems disease)

APPENDIX NINE

Glossary of Terms

Acropachy. "Clubbing" of the fingers with thickening of skin at the base of the nails, often with an increase in the curvature of the nails. Acropachy is very occasionally seen in patients with Graves' disease.

AIDS. Acquired immunodeficiency syndrome.

Ambidexterity. Partial left-handedness.

Amiodarone. A heart drug that contains a large amount of iodine. Amiodarone can cause abnormal thyroid function.

Anaplastic cancer. A very malignant form of thyroid cancer.

Antigen. Any substance that has the capacity to induce an immune response.

Antigen-presenting cell. A cell involved in the immune process.

Antiperoxidose (antimicrosomal) antibody. Antibody directed against peroxidose, a protein located in tiny particles known as microsomes within thyroid cells.

Apathetic hyperthyroidism. A type of thyroid overactivity seen in elderly patients, with so few symptoms and signs that the thyroid problem is often unrecognized.

Artificial tears. Eyedrops used to lubricate dry eyes.

Attention deficit disorder. A type of learning disability in which the individual has difficulty concentrating on particular tasks.

Autoantibody. Antibody directed against one's own tissues.

Beta-adrenergic receptors. Receptors on the cell surface that bind adrenaline, a hormone that can cause rapid heartbeat, tremor, and nervousness.

Beta-blockers. A class of drugs that block "beta-adrenergic receptors" and are capable of diminishing many symp-

231

toms of thyroid-hormone excess. Propranolol, atenolol, metoprolol, and nadolol are all beta-blocking drugs.

Biliary cirrhosis. A condition in which bile flow is impeded, leading to liver damage.

Bipolar disease. A form of depression in which the mood cycles between exhilaration and depression.

Bone-density test. A test that evaluates the calcium content of bone, used to diagnose osteoporosis.

Calcitonin. A hormone made by C cells in the thyroid, which helps regulate calcium.

Carpal tunnel syndrome. A neurological condition in which compression of an important nerve at the wrist (the median nerve) may cause hand weakness, numbness, and pain.

Cassava. A plant that has a high level of thiocyanate, which can cause goiter, especially in areas of the world where there is also iodine deficiency.

CAT scan. A special X ray procedure, sometimes used to evaluate the size or location of the thyroid, thyroid eye problems, or thyroid tumors.

Chernobyl. Site of the 1986 nuclear accident in the Ukraine.

Click murmur. A sound commonly caused by mitral valve prolapse.

Cold nodule. A nonfunctioning thyroid lump that does not concentrate radioactive isotopes in a thyroid scan.

Cretinism. Permanent physical and mental impairment due to severe thyroid deficiency in early life.

Crohn's disease. A disease in which the small intestine is inflamed.

Curie. A measure of radiation. A millicurie is $\frac{1}{1000}$th of a Curie.

Cytokine. A type of protein hormone involved in the immune process.

Cytoplasm. The part of a cell surrounding the nucleus.

Cytotoxic. Having the ability to destroy another cell.

Dulse. Seaweed.

Echocardiogram. A heart test in which ultrasound is used to study the anatomy and function of the heart.

Electromyogram (EMG). A test done to evaluate muscle function.

Endemic hypothyroidism. A place where thyroid deficiency is commonly found, often due to iodine deficiency.

Fallout. Radioactive material that falls from the sky after a nuclear accident contaminating the environment, including crops and water supplies.

Fine needle aspiration. A type of thyroid biopsy using a very thin needle.

Follicular cancer. A type of thyroid cancer.

Free thyroid hormone level. Active or "unbound" hormone that reacts with body tissues.

Generalized resistance to thyroid hormone (GRTH). A condition in which body cells respond subnormally to thyroid hormone, due to abnormal thyroid hormone receptors.

Goiter belt. Part of the midwestern United States surrounding the Great Lakes where iodine-deficiency goiter was a common occurrence until the introduction of iodized salt in the mid-1920s.

Goitrogen. A substance that may cause the thyroid to enlarge, forming a goiter.

Human chorionic gonadatropin (HCG). A placental hormone that helps maintain pregnancy in the early months of gestation.

Hürthle cell cancer. A form of thyroid cancer.

Immunoglobulin. Proteins that function as antibodies.

Interferon gamma. A protein able to inhibit viral activity.

Interleukin-1 (IL-1). A protein induced by macrophages and T cells in an immune reaction.

Kombu. Seaweed.

Lupus Erythematosis. An immune disease in which antibodies are made to many different types of body cells.

Lymphocytic hypophysitis. Inflammation of the pituitary gland.

Macrophage. A scavenger cell that is very important in activating the immune system.

Major histocompatibility complex (MHC). Cell-membrane receptors that bind to antigens and thus help initiate immune reactions.

Median nerve. An important nerve supplying sensation and strength to the hand.

Medullary cancer. A type of thyroid cancer involving a specialized type of thyroid cell known as the C cell because it manufactures calcitonin. Medullary cancer may be hereditary.

Mitral valve prolapse (MVP). A heart condition due to improper closure of one of the heart valves.

Multiple sclerosis. An autoimmune inflammatory condition of the nervous system.

Neonatal hyperthyroidism. Overactivity of the thyroid in a newborn.

Nonsteroidal anti-inflammatory drug (NSAID). A group of drugs that reduce inflammation. Examples are Advil (ibuprofen), Motrin, Naprosyn, and Indomethacin.

Nucleus. A central part of the cell that contains genetic material that controls cell functions. The nucleus also contains the thyroid-hormone receptor.

Oncogene. A gene found in all cells that may help convert normal cells to cancer cells.

Oophoritis. Inflammation of the ovaries.

Orbital decompression. Eye surgery involving removal of part of the bony orbit to reduce eye protrusion.

Osteoporosis. A condition characterized especially by bone loss from the hip and spine, with increased risk for fractures.

Papillary cancer. The commonest form of thyroid cancer.

Parathyroid. Glands usually located behind the thyroid that control calcium and bone metabolism.

Periodic paralysis. Intermittent, partial, or total loss of strength due to shifts in potassium into cells rarely seen in Graves' disease, especially in Asian men.

Petechiae. Small red spots due to tiny hemorrhages within the skin.

Platelets. Small blood cells that have an important role in blood clotting.

Postpartum depression. Depression after pregnancy.

Postpartum thyroiditis. Thyroid inflammation occurring after pregnancy.

Potassium iodide. A drug used to treat certain thyroid disorders. It can also be used to block the uptake by the thyroid of radioactive-iodine isotopes that are released in a nuclear-reactor accident.

Radioisotope. A radioactive substance that emits specific kinds of radiation. Radioisotopes of iodine are used for thyroid scans and thyroid therapy.

Raynaud's syndrome. A disorder caused by spasm of tiny arteries in the hands and feet often brought on by cold temperatures.

Receptor. A special site on the cell surface or within the cell where specific chemicals, especially hormones, bind and initiate a variety of actions within the target cell.

Regional enteritis. A synonym for Crohn's disease.

Schirmer test. A test done to evaluate tearing of the eyes.

Scleroderma. An immune disorder affecting many parts of the body including particularly the skin and the intestine.

Selenium. A trace element used by thyroid cells that may help protect against diseases due to iodine deficiency.

Silent thyroiditis. Painless thyroiditis.

Sjögren's syndrome. An immune condition leading to a decrease in tearing, saliva production, and vaginal secretions.

Subclinical hyperthyroidism. Mild thyroid overactivity unaccompanied by obvious symptoms or physical signs.

Subclinical hypothyroidism. Mild thyroid underactivity unaccompanied by obvious symptoms or physical signs.

Substernal goiter. A goiter located under the breastbone.

T cell. A type of lymphocyte involved in cellular immunity.

  Helper T Cell. A lymphocyte involved in cellular immunity.

  Suppresser T Cell. A lymphocyte that tends to decrease immune activity.

  Killer T Cell. Lymphocytes that can destroy invading antigenic cells or normal body tissues in certain autoimmune diseases.

  Natural killer cell. Lymphocytes that can destroy invading antigenic cells or normal body tissues in certain autoimmune diseases.

  Cytotoxic T cell. Lymphocytes that can destroy invading antigenic cells or normal body tissues in certain autoimmune diseases.

Thiocyanate. A chemical found in some foods that may interfere with thyroid function.

Three Mile Island. Site of a minor nuclear accident in Pennsylvania.

Thrombocytopenic purpura. A condition in which platelets are reduced in number and that may lead to bleeding disorders.

Thyroglobulin. A protein in the thyroid in which thyroid hormones are manufactured and stored. Some thyroglobulin is secreted into the blood stream and can be used as a marker for the presence of thyroid disease, especially thyroid cancer.

Thyroiditis. Thyroid inflammation. There are several forms of thyroiditis, including chronic or Hashimoto's thyroiditis, subacute thyroiditis, and painless or postpartum thyroiditis.

Ulcerative colitis. An illness in which the large intestine (colon) becomes inflamed.

Index